Regina Furlong Lind, MSW, LCSW
Debra Honig Bachman, MSW, LCSW
Editors

Fundamentals of Perinatal Social Work: A Guide for Clinical Practice with Women, Infants, and Families

Pre-publication
REVIEWS,
COMMENTARIES,
EVALUATIONS . . .

"**T**his Handbook is a knowledgeable summation of the essence of perinatal social work that is long overdue. It is a must for any beginning perinatal social worker to own one!"

Charlotte Collins Bursi, MSSW
Perinatal Social Worker
University of Tennessee Newborn Center
Memphis, TN
Founding President
National Association
of Perinatal Social Workers

More pre-publication
REVIEWS, COMMENTARIES, EVALUATIONS . . .

"**A** long-needed resource for students and social workers entering perinatal practice, *Fundamentals of Perinatal Social Work . . .* not only provides an overview of topics pertinent to the field but also has sufficient depth to serve as an ongoing reference for practice.

In recent years perinatal social work has expanded beyond the boundaries of the hospital NICU and OB services; we now find perinatal social workers practicing in HIV treatment settings, public and home health services, technology-assisted reproduction, and other areas. This publication should serve as an invaluable tool to those seeking to broaden their knowledge base in response to the changing needs of patients and families in the perinatal period."

Brenda C. Sumrall, MSW
Director of Social Work
and Instructor in Pediatrics
(Social Work)
University Hospitals and Clinics
The University of Mississippi
Medical Center

"**P**erinatal social workers will find *Fundamentals of Perinatal Social Work: A Guide for Clinical Practice with Women, Infants, and Families* to be a valuable resource for our work with women, infants, and families.

The authors and editors are respected, well-seasoned perinatal social workers. They are my colleagues and many have been my mentors as I set out to learn this specialized field of practice 17 years ago.

The time before, during, and after birth brings great joy, immense sorrow, and a multiplicity of changes and growth for families. My colleagues will welcome this book, and our clients will be the better for our shared knowledge."

Joni Hardcastle, MSW
Perinatal Social Worker
Group Health Cooperative
of Puget Sound
Seattle, WA
Member and Past President
National Association
of Perinatal Social Workers

The Haworth Press, Inc.

Fundamentals
of Perinatal Social Work:
A Guide for Clinical Practice
with Women, Infants,
and Families

Fundamentals
of Perinatal Social Work:
A Guide for Clinical Practice
with Women, Infants,
and Families

Regina Furlong Lind, MSW, LCSW
Debra Honig Bachman, MSW, LCSW
Editors

The Haworth Press, Inc.
New York • London

Fundamentals of Perinatal Social Work: A Guide for Clinical Practice with Women, Infants, and Families has also been published as *Social Work in Health Care*, Volume 24, Numbers 3/4 1997.

The development, preparation, and publication of this work has been undertaken with great care. However, the publisher, employees, editors, and agents of The Haworth Press and all imprints of The Haworth Press, Inc., including The Haworth Medical Press and Pharmaceutical Products Press, are not responsible for any errors contained herein or for consequences that may ensue from use of materials or information contained in this work. Opinions expressed by the author(s) are not necessarily those of The Haworth Press, Inc.

The Haworth Press, Inc., 10 Alice Street, Binghamton, NY 13904-1580 USA

Library of Congress Cataloging-in-Publication Data

Fundamentals of perinatal social work: a guide for clinical practice with women, infants, and families/Regina Furlong Lind, Debra Honig Bachman, editors.
    p. cm.
    "Has also been published as Social work in health care, volume 24, numbers 3/4 1997."
    Includes bibliographical references and index.
    ISBN 0-7890-0043-1 (alk. paper).–ISBN 0-7890-0049-0 (pbk.: alk. paper)
    1. Maternal and infant welfare–United States. 2. Medical social work–United States. I. Lind, Regina Furlong. II. Bachman, Debra Honig.
HV699.F86 1997
362.1'0425–dc21   97-6350
                                                               CIP

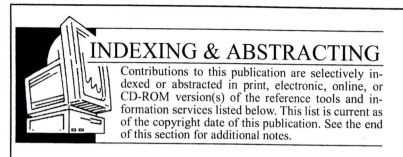

INDEXING & ABSTRACTING

Contributions to this publication are selectively indexed or abstracted in print, electronic, online, or CD-ROM version(s) of the reference tools and information services listed below. This list is current as of the copyright date of this publication. See the end of this section for additional notes.

- *Abstracts in Social Gerontology: Current Literature on Aging*, National Council on the Aging, Library, 409 Third Street SW, 2nd Floor, Washington, DC 20024

- *Academic Abstracts/CD-ROM*, EBSCO Publishing Editorial Department, P.O. Box 590, Ipswich, MA 01938-0590

- *Applied Social Sciences Index & Abstracts (ASSIA) (Online: ASSI via Data-Star) (CDRom: ASSIA Plus)*, Bowker-Saur Limited, Maypole House, Maypole Road, East Grinstead, West Sussex RH19 1HH, England

- *Behavioral Medicine Abstracts*, The Society of Behavioral Medicine, 103 South Adams Street, Rockville, MD 20850

- *caredata CD: the social and community care database*, National Institute for Social Work, 5 Tavistock Place, London WC1H 9SS, England

- *CINAHL (Cumulative Index to Nursing & Allied Health Literature), in print, also on CD-ROM from CD PLUS, EBSCO, and SilverPlatter, and online from CDP Online (formerly BRS), Data-Star, and PaperChase. (Support materials include Subject Heading List, Database Search Guide, and instructional video.)*, CINAHL Information Systems, P.O. Box 871/1509 Wilson Terrace, Glendale, CA 91209-0871

- *CNPIEC Reference Guide: Chinese National Directory of Foreign Periodicals*, P.O. Box 88, Beijing, People's Republic of China

(continued)

- **Communication Abstracts**, Temple University, 303 Annenberg Hall, Philadelphia, PA 19122

- **Current Contents . . . . see: Institute for Scientific Information**

- **Excerpta Medica/Secondary Publishing Division**, Elsevier Science Inc., Secondary Publishing Division, 655 Avenue of the Americas, New York, NY 10010

- **Family Studies Database (online and CD/ROM)**, National Information Services Corporation, 306 East Baltimore Pike, 2nd Floor, Media, PA 19063

- **Health Source: Indexing & Abstracting of 160 selected health related journals, updated monthly**, EBSCO Publishing, 83 Pine Street, Peabody, MA 01960

- **Health Source Plus: expanded version of "Health Source" to be released shortly**, EBSCO Publishing, 83 Pine Street, Peabody, MA 01960

- **Hospital and Health Administration Index**, American Hospital Association, One North Franklin, Chicago, IL 60606

- **Human Resources Abstracts (HRA)**, Sage Publications, Inc., 2455 Teller Road, Newbury Park, CA 91320

- **IBZ International Bibliography of Periodical Literature**, Zeller Verlag GmbH & Co., P.O.B. 1949, D-49009 Osnabruck, Germany

- **Index Medicus**, NATIONAL LIBRARY OF MEDICINE, 8600 Rockville Pike, Bethesda, MD 20894

- **Index to Periodical Articles Related to Law**, University of Texas, 727 East 26th Street, Austin, TX 78705

- **Institute for Scientific Information**, 3501 Market Street, Philadelphia, PA 19104-3302 USA. Coverage in:
  a) Social Science Citation Index (SSCI): print, online, CD-ROM
  b) Research Alert (current awareness service)
  c) Social SciSearch (magnetic tape)
  d) Current Contents/Social & Behavioral Sciences (weekly current awareness service)

(continued)

- *INTERNET ACCESS (& additional networks) Bulletin Board for Libraries ("BUBL"), coverage of information resources on INTERNET, JANET, and other networks.*
  - JANET X.29: UK.AC.BATH.BUBL or 00006012101300
  - TELNET: BUBL.BATH.AC.UK or 138.38.32.45 login 'bubl'
  - Gopher: BUBL.BATH.AC.UK (138.32.32.45). Port 7070
  - World Wide Web: http: / / www.bubl.bath.ac.uk./BUBL/ home.html
  - NISSWAIS: telnetniss.ac.uk (for the NISS gateway)
  The Andersonian Library, Curran Building, 101 St James Road, Glasgow G4 0NS, Scotland

- *Psychological Abstracts (PsycINFO)*, American Psychological Association, P.O. Box 91600, Washington, DC 20090-1600

- *Referativnyi Zhurnal (Abstracts Journal of the Institute of Scientific Information of the Republic of Russia)*, The Institute of Scientific Information, Baltijskaja ul., 14, Moscow A-219, Republic of Russia

- *Social Planning/Policy & Development Abstracts (SOPODA)*, Sociological Abstracts, Inc., P.O. Box 22206, San Diego, CA 92192-0206

- *Social Science Citation Index . . . . see: Institute for Scientific Information*

- *Social Work Abstracts*, National Association of Social Workers, 750 First Street NW, 8th Floor, Washington, DC 20002

- *Sociological Abstracts (SA)*, Sociological Abstracts, Inc., P.O. Box 22206, San Diego, CA 92192-0206

- *SOMED (social medicine) Database*, Landes Institut fur Den Offentlichen Gesundheitsdienst NRW, Postfach 20 10 12, D-33548 Bielefeld, Germany

- *Special Educational Needs Abstracts*, Carfax Information Systems, P.O. Box 25, Abingdon, Oxfordshire OX14 3UE, United Kingdom

(continued)

- **Studies on Women Abstracts**, Carfax Publishing Company, P.O. Box 25, Abingdon, Oxfordshire OX14 3UE, United Kingdom

- **Violence and Abuse Abstracts: A Review of Current Literature on Interpersonal Violence (VAA)**, Sage Publications, Inc., 2455 Teller Road, Newbury Park, CA 91320

SPECIAL BIBLIOGRAPHIC NOTES

related to special journal issues (separates)
and indexing/abstracting

☐ indexing/abstracting services in this list will also cover material in any "separate" that is co-published simultaneously with Haworth's special thematic journal issue or DocuSerial. Indexing/abstracting usually covers material at the article/chapter level.

☐ monographic co-editions are intended for either non-subscribers or libraries which intend to purchase a second copy for their circulating collections.

☐ monographic co-editions are reported to all jobbers/wholesalers/approval plans. The source journal is listed as the "series" to assist the prevention of duplicate purchasing in the same manner utilized for books-in-series.

☐ to facilitate user/access services all indexing/abstracting services are encouraged to utilize the co-indexing entry note indicated at the bottom of the first page of each article/chapter/contribution.

☐ this is intended to assist a library user of any reference tool (whether print, electronic, online, or CD-ROM) to locate the monographic version if the library has purchased this version but not a subscription to the source journal.

☐ individual articles/chapters in any Haworth publication are also available through the Haworth Document Delivery Services (HDDS).

Fundamentals of Perinatal Social Work: A Guide for Clinical Practice with Women, Infants, and Families

CONTENTS

ABOUT THE EDITORS

Regina Furlong Lind, MSW, LCSW, retired from private practice of social work in 1990. She is a current member and former Associate Chair of the Illinois Chapter of Committee on Inquiry of the National Association of Social Workers and former Chair of the Standards Committee of the National Association of Perinatal Social Workers. Prior to private practice, Ms. Lind worked as a Clinical Social Worker and supervisor in the newborn intensive care units and social work departments in hospitals in Kentucky, Connecticut, and Illinois. She is the co-author of numerous articles on perinatal loss, prenatal diagnosis, and neonatal intensive care.

Debra Honig Bachman, MSW, LCSW, is a Clinical Social Worker at the University of Illinois Medical Center in Chicago, a position she previously held at the Children's Memorial Medical Center, also in Chicago. She is co-founder and co-president of Chicago Hadassah's Council for Social Workers & Related Mental Health Professionals and former co-president of the Association of Pediatric Social Workers. Ms. Bachman has been a member of the National Association of Social Workers since 1990.

The editors wish to thank the National Association of Perinatal Social Work for their support in this project.

Introduction

Ruth Lyall Breslin, MSW, LCSW

When the first full-time social worker was assigned to the Newborn Special Care Unit for premature and sick infants at Yale-New Haven Hospital in 1964, it marked the formal beginning of the field of practice that we now know as perinatal social work. Evolving along with advances in medical treatment of mother, fetus, and newborn, the development of this new area of service was informed by traditional social work practices and concerns, and influenced by the larger historical context of social changes taking place in the United States during the 1960s and 1970s.

The philosophical and theoretical underpinnings of social work practice focus on the individual in the context of their social unit. This philosophical stance led hospital social workers to an early and still evolving concern with identifying and promoting a healthy social and emotional environment for pregnant women and/or infants long before medicine had the scientific and technological ability to take a parallel look at the maternal-fetal physiological environment.

Similarly, early social work interest in both the acute and chronic effect of disease and injury on individuals, families, and communities laid the foundation for perinatal social work's commitment to and expertise in providing both short- and long-term supportive interventions to individuals and families in crisis. In short, although the official development of perinatal social work may have begun in 1964, its roots go back to 1905 when the first hospital social workers began to practice at Massachusetts General Hospital.

Ruth Lyall Breslin is now retired as Director of Social Work at the Yale New Haven Hospital and as Assistant Clinical Professor in the Department of Obstetrics/Gynecology and Pediatrics, Yale University School of Medicine. Mrs. Breslin was the first social worker in the original Newborn Special Care Unit at Yale.

[Haworth co-indexing entry note]: "Introduction." Breslin, Ruth Lyall. Co-published simultaneously in *Social Work in Health Care* (The Haworth Press, Inc.) Vol. 24, No. 3/4, 1997, pp. 1-2; and: *Fundamentals of Perinatal Social Work: A Guide for Clinical Practice with Women, Infants, and Families* (ed: Regina Furlong Lind, and Debra Honig Bachman) The Haworth Press, Inc., 1997, pp. 1-2. Single or multiple copies of this article are available for a fee from The Haworth Document Delivery Service [1-800-342-9678, 9:00 a.m. - 5:00 p.m. (EST). E-mail address: getinfo@haworth.com].

1

Perinatal social work today, associated as it is with a rapidly advancing and technologically sophisticated area of medicine, has an easily understood reputation for innovation. After all, perinatal medicine developed in the space of 10 years as its initial focus on the care of the neonate expanded to encompass maternal-fetal care. Social work was an integral part of that development from the beginning so it is certainly understandable that perinatal social work has been seen and sees itself as breaking new ground.

This special volume, with its focus on the field of Perinatal Social Work, is the culmination of work begun in 1992 in conjunction with and supported by the National Association of Perinatal Social Work. The first two articles were originally written by Ms. Debra Honig Bachman during her field placement as a handbook for new perinatal social workers. Often students and new workers find themselves overwhelmed with the medical information and technology they must understand in order to function in their position. As is so often the case with social work practice in a host setting, the literature which guides the social work practice is shared, in this case with medicine, nursing, public health and others. The new worker must gather a body of literature to use as a reference in his or her work. While this is an interesting and stimulating exercise, it is one a busy student or a new worker may not have the luxury of doing.

The articles which follow will provide such a reference and illustrate the depth and breadth the field of Perinatal Social Work has come to encompass today. Perinatal Social Workers are no longer employed only in hospital settings but work in AIDS Clinics, Public Health settings, Ethics Centers, and Private Practice. However, what has not changed is the goal to maximize the potential of every infant and every family–the true art of healing–in the future.

Perinatal Social Work
and the High Risk Obstetrics Patient

Debra Honig Bachman, MSW, LCSW
Regina Furlong Lind, MSW, LCSW

SUMMARY. Even under the most favorable conditions, pregnancy and childbirth may tax the family's ability to cope. If there are problems with the pregnancy, these coping capacities may be further stressed. This article examines the common high risk obstetrical problems, frequently seen emotional reactions to the treatment of those problems, and social work assessment and intervention with families. *[Article copies available for a fee from The Haworth Document Delivery Service: 1-800-342-9678. E-mail address: getinfo@haworth.com]*

CRISIS THEORY, PREGNANCY,
AND THE HIGH RISK PREGNANCY

Few events in the developmental life of the family have as strong an impact as the addition of a new member(s) through pregnancy and childbirth. Even though families plan and anticipate such additions, the pregnancy and delivery may precipitate a "disruption in the normal state of equilibrium" (Parad, 1965), also known as a crisis.

The authors wish to acknowledge the work of Ms. Rebecca Pruitt whose invaluable guidance, encouragement, and support played a major role in developing the original format of this project. Without her dynamic teaching and solid knowledge base of perinatal social work, this project would not have been possible.

[Haworth co-indexing entry note]: "Perinatal Social Work and the High Risk Obstetrics Patient." Bachman, Debra Honig, and Regina Furlong Lind. Co-published simultaneously in *Social Work in Health Care* (The Haworth Press, Inc.) Vol. 24, No. 3/4, 1997, pp. 3-19; and: *Fundamentals of Perinatal Social Work: A Guide for Clinical Practice with Women, Infants, and Families* (ed: Regina Furlong Lind, and Debra Honig Bachman) The Haworth Press, Inc., 1997, pp. 3-19. Single or multiple copies of this article are available for a fee from The Haworth Document Delivery Service [1-800-342-9678, 9:00 a.m. - 5:00 p.m. (EST). E-mail address: getinfo@ haworth.com].

Bibring (1959) was one of the first to document the intense emotional and physical stresses pregnancy and childbirth precipitate. She writes, "Pregnancy, like puberty and menopause is regarded as a period of crisis involving profound endocrine and general somatic as well as psychological changes."

As with other maturational crises, certain tasks must be mastered in order for the individual/family to develop and move on to new levels of functioning. Several authors describe the tasks which expectant families must master in order to successfully love and nurture their developing babies. These tasks include: accepting the reality of the pregnancy, attaching to the developing fetus, negotiating changes in family relationships, preparing to parent the baby, and developing a reality-based relationship with the baby (Bibring et al., 1961; Shields, 1974).

In most cases, pregnancies develop normally and despite the great physical and emotional demands, families master the tasks set before them, mature and grow. In some instances, physical or medical problems may prevent or complicate pregnancy. When this occurs, families need medical and psychosocial intervention to help them maintain their equilibrium, continue to meet the challenges presented to them and avoid being overwhelmed by stress.

The medical/psychosocial intervention is usually provided by a perinatal health care team in a High Risk Pregnancy Unit of a hospital. (The term perinatal refers to the 60 days around the time of delivery.) The Perinatal Social Worker is an essential member of the health care team who provides services to families experiencing a range of reproductive problems including infertility, pregnancy termination as a result of prenatal diagnosis, HIV, adoption, chemical dependency, and fetal loss. This article, however, will focus on the limits of its scope to work with families with medical complications. We begin by describing the common medical problems and the emotional reaction to high risk pregnancy. Then we will explore the Perinatal Social Worker's assessment and intervention.

COMMON PERINATAL MEDICAL PROBLEMS

Complications may occur at any time during pregnancy. They may be life threatening to the mother and/or baby, or may be fairly benign, requiring little intervention. Most often, however, complications of pregnancy require maternal hospitalization, even if just for evaluation. After evaluation, some patients may be treated outside of the hospital. The social worker on the perinatal unit must be familiar with the most frequent pregnancy complications and the implications for patients, families, and the hospital staff who treat them. The following are brief descriptions of the most common complications, preceded by a short discussion of infertility. Though infertility is not a complication of pregnancy, it is a common perinatal problem.

Infertility

Infertility is defined as the inability to conceive despite at least one year of unprotected sexual intercourse and/or the inability to carry a pregnancy to live birth. Fifteen to twenty percent of Americans who try to conceive are considered infertile. The etiology of infertility is varied and the problem is seen among males and females alike. Common causes for female infertility include scarring of the fallopian tubes or ovaries from previous infections (pelvic inflammatory disease, sexually transmitted diseases, infections from IUD's), endometriosis, endocrine problems, structural problems in the uterus, or genetic abnormalities. Common causes for male infertility include complications in sperm production from past infections, environmental factors, blockage of sperm from tissue scarring, or dysfunction in sperm delivery (Batterman, 1985; Greenfeld et al., 1988; Shapiro, 1986).

The impact of infertility affects individuals as any other loss and a period of mourning follows its diagnosis. This mourning also manifests itself after each failed attempt to conceive. Many couples mourn month after month while attempting to achieve pregnancy. Such a mourning period is also common among couples who conceive but later miscarry one, or more times (Batterman, 1985; Greenfeld et al., 1988; Shapiro, 1986).

Hyperemesis Gravidarum

This condition is characterized by severe, persistent vomiting which continues beyond the 12th week of pregnancy and usually ends by the 28th week. The patient may experience dehydration, weight loss, reduced food intake, electrolyte and vitamin deficiency, anemia and increased acidity to the arterial blood. Treatment includes bedrest, hospitalization, rehydration, electrolyte replenishment, restricted food intake, and medications to manage the vomiting. If this treatment is unsuccessful, it may be necessary to administer nutrition through hyperalimentation, an intravenous fluid which supplies nutritional needs. There is not one known cause for this condition, though it has been postulated that it may be due to a hormone imbalance (Connon, 1995).

Placenta Previa

In this condition the placenta is abnormally placed low over the cervix, the opening to the birth canal (Harrison, 1983; Naeye & Tafari, 1983;

Pilliteri, 1992). The cervix may be either totally covered (Total placenta previa) or only partially covered (Partial placenta previa) (Harrison, 1983; Pilliteri, 1992). During the second half of pregnancy, the placenta may become partially displaced and bleeding may occur. If this occurs, the patient may require total bedrest. Patients with placenta previa usually deliver by Cesarean section (Pilliteri, 1992; Resnick & Moore, 1995).

Though one clear cause has not been identified, the following may be associated with placenta previa: multigravida pregnancy, previous Cesarean sections, advanced maternal age, poor uterine circulation, uterine scarring, fibroids, multiple gestation pregnancy, tobacco or cocaine use during pregnancy and living at high altitudes (Berger et al., 1990; Giacoia, 1990; Harrison, 1983; Naeye & Tafari, 1983; Pilliteri, 1992).

Premature Rupture of Membranes (PROM)

This condition, which may occur any time during pregnancy, is characterized by the rupture of the membranes surrounding the fetus, resulting in loss of amniotic fluid (Harrison, 1983; Pilliteri, 1992). Many patients with PROM deliver prematurely but, in the absence of any evidence of compromise to the fetus' health, efforts are made to allow the fetus to remain in the uterus to optimize its healthy growth and development. The patients who do deliver shortly after the rupture occurs usually do so because infection develops, and labor cannot and should not be stopped (Johnson & Daikoku, 1985; Pilliteri, 1992). PROM puts the fetus at high risk for fetal hypoxia (insufficient oxygen), meconium (waste) aspiration, respiratory distress, hypoplastic lung (insufficient development of lung tissue) and infection (Resnick & Moore, 1995).

PROM often occurs in patients with multiple gestation pregnancy, low pregnancy weight gain, premature opening of an incompetent cervix, polyhydramnios (excess of amniotic fluid), cervical surgeries prior to pregnancy, and use of "crack" cocaine or tobacco during pregnancy. Advanced maternal age, recent coitus, obesity, stand-up work during pregnancy, and placenta previa are often associated with PROM (Giacoia, 1990; Harrison, 1983; Naeye & Tafari, 1983; Pilliteri, 1992).

Some studies have postulated that PROM may be caused by acute infection. The infection, they theorize, triggers the release of an enzyme which in turn brings about changes in the membrane, causing its rupture (Johnson & Daikoku, 1985; Pilliteri, 1992).

Pregnancy Induced Hypertension (PIH)

PIH describes elevated blood pressure, usually occurring before the 24th week of gestation, and may accompany more severe symptoms

(Pilliteri, 1992; Roberts, 1989). There are several types of PIH including PIH superimposed on women with preexisting hypertension, mild to severe Preeclampsia, and Eclampsia (Roberts, 1989; Worley, 1986). When albumin (protein in the urine) and edema are present in PIH, the patient is said to have Preeclampsia (Pilliteri, 1992; Roberts, 1989; Worley, 1986).

Some PIH patients develop seizures, convulsions and/or coma. This more serious and potentially life-threatening condition is referred to as Eclampsia. Some believe that Eclampsia is preventable if PIH is managed well in the early, less severe stages (Roberts, 1989). Predisposing factors to PIH include first time pregnancy, age (between 20-30 years of age), low socioeconomic level, Diabetic history, women who have had 5 or more pregnancies, polyhydramnios, multiple gestation pregnancy, and hypertensive cardiovascular disease (Pilliteri, 1992; Roberts, 1989).

Patients with PIH often have poor blood circulation to the uterus, resulting in a fetus which is small for gestational age (S.G.A.). During pregnancy, hospitalization, bedrest and blood pressure medications are often prescribed to control symptoms, though sometimes labor must be induced for the safety of mother and child (Harrison, 1983; Pilliteri, 1992; Worley, 1986).

Premature Labor

Premature labor is labor occurring between the end of the 20th and the 37th weeks of gestation (Benson, 1986; Pilliteri, 1992; Resnick & Moore, 1995). Predisposing factors may include lack of prenatal care or nutrition, severe emotional distress, age (under 17 or over 40), low socioeconomic status, employment activity level and history of preterm labor (Benson, 1986; Pilliteri, 1992; Resnick & Moore, 1995). However, premature labor may occur in the absence of these factors. Premature labor may be precipitated by other perinatal complications including PIH, urinary tract infections, uterine abnormalities, placenta previa, polyhydramnios and multiple gestation pregnancies (Manginello & DiGeronimo, 1991). In addition, maternal surgical procedures during pregnancy, trauma and chronic medical conditions such as Cardiovascular disease, renal disease, severe anemia, cholestatis of pregnancy, or Diabetes are also related to premature labor (Benson, 1986; Pilliteri, 1992; Resnick & Moore, 1995).

Most women with premature labor are hospitalized, medicated, and confined to bed in an attempt to decrease uterine contractions. Tocolytics, or drugs prescribed to control preterm labor, include terbutaline, ritodrine and isoxsuprine (Benson, 1986; Harrison, 1983; Pilliteri, 1992; Resnick & Moore, 1995). Home care may involve complex, high tech medical intervention such as monitors to record contractions, or infusion pumps to administer tocolytic medications (Pilliteri, 1992; Resnick & Moore, 1995).

Despite the use of medical technology, many patients who experience preterm labor deliver early (Harrison, 1983; Pilliteri, 1992). The premature infant is usually admitted to the NICU and may experience complications associated with early birth such as Respiratory Distress Syndrome, Patent Ductus Arteriosis, and Intraventricular Hemorrhage.

Diabetes

This common metabolic disorder alters the way the body breaks down and utilizes glucose. As pregnancy also affects the balance of the metabolic system, the pregnant diabetic and her developing child may be at increased risk for metabolic problems. For the pregnant perinatal patient, a goal of medical treatment is to maintain an adequate level of insulin, a hormone produced by the pancreas which converts glucose to energy to maintain optimal health of mother and child (Buchanan & Coustan, 1995; Kitzmiller et al., 1982).

Diabetes may be diagnosed pre-gestationally or during pregnancy. Among pre-gestation diabetics, some do not produce insulin and require injections while others make insulin but need medical attention to properly utilize it (Buchanan & Coustan, 1995). Gestational Diabetes may develop between the 24th and 28th weeks of gestation. These patients may be managed by diet while others require insulin injections. Many (perhaps 50-60%) of these patients resume normoglycemia following delivery, but may develop the condition again later in their lives (Buchanan & Coustan, 1995).

The patient who has been diabetic since her youth is familiar with the procedure for injecting insulin. Her past functioning is usually a predictor of how well she will deal with her Diabetes while pregnant. The woman who develops Gestational Diabetes and needs insulin supplements, however, must make a major lifestyle adaptation. These changes often precipitate feelings of sadness, anger, frustration and loss of control. Increased separation from family due to frequent perinatal hospitalizations and fear about her own health and the health of the fetus are also common emotional issues (Furlong Lind & Beck Black, 1988).

Complications of pregnancy seen in diabetic women include hypertension, anemia, proteinuria, hemorrhage, coronary artery disease and retinopathies. Further, diabetic perinatal patients tend to deliver large babies. As delivery of large babies can be complicated, labor is sometimes induced between 35 and 38 weeks of gestation. However, early delivery may precipitate the development of problems of prematurity such as Respiratory Distress Syndrome. Other medical problems among infants of diabetic mothers include hypoglycemia, hyperbilirubinemia, hypocalcemia, poor feeding, multiple congenital anomalies including anencephaly, spina bifida, hydrocephalus, and malformations of the cardiac, anal/rectal or renal systems. Prenatal treatment of the insulin dependent diabetic emphasizes the importance of maintaining normal blood sugars to minimize birth defects which may occur and have a bearing on healthy development of the fetus (Kitzmiller et al., 1982).

Multiple Gestation

All multiple gestations are considered high risk because of increased likelihood of maternal hypertension, polyhydramnios, anemia, placenta previa, postpartum hemorrhage and premature labor and delivery. The fetus is also at risk for birth defects or poor growth. In addition, the incidence of premature labor and delivery increases with the number of fetuses in the uterus. The majority of multiple gestation neonates are admitted to the NICU as they tend to be small and/or premature (Harrison, 1983; Killam & Trofatter, 1986; Manginello & DiGeronimo, 1991; Pilliteri, 1992).

Often patients with multiple gestation are admitted to the hospital if they are medically unstable for any reason. These patients usually express marked anxiety when discussing the impending birth of multiples. This anxiety is related to the viability and well-being of the babies, ability to care for several babies at once, and financial concerns. It is important that parents be allowed to express these fears and reservations as they may be surrounded by family and friends who are emphasizing the novelty and uniqueness of the experience rather than the enormous risk and responsibility.

Occasionally, one or more of the fetuses may die prior to delivery (intrauterine fetal demise: IUFD). The demise of a fetus is particularly common among pregnancies with three or more fetuses (Killam & Trofatter, 1986). Often parents know about such a loss prior to delivery through routine ultrasound examination. Special attention and support should be given to parents who experience such a loss as they may be told by well-meaning individuals that they should be happy for the surviving children and not grieve. While this may ultimately be true, parents may need to mourn the infant(s) lost before continuing to bond with the survivors.

In gestations where there are three or more fetuses, fetal reduction may be offered as an option to parents. Multi-fetal reduction refers to a procedure done in the first trimester of pregnancy in which one or more fetuses are terminated, "with no knowledge of any fetal characteristics" (Berkowitz & Lynch, 1990). The purpose of this procedure is to maximize the safe inutero growth of the remaining fetuses.

Parents who choose this option need special support and attention.

They may feel guilt and grief related to the lost fetuses yet at the same time express hope for the remaining ones (Schreiner-Engel et al., 1995; Walther, 1990). Since many of these patients are previously infertile, the irony of having to make such a decision may be especially painful.

Prenatal Diagnosis and Fetal Therapy

Prenatal diagnosis, or the use of medical procedures to detect or rule out genetic and/or congenital anomalies in the fetus, was introduced in the 1960s, when amniocentesis was first used to remove and test amniotic fluid. Since that time the types of testing and the ability to diagnose disorders has increased rapidly as has the ability to treat certain fetal problems inutero. The use of sophisticated ultrasound equipment and the ability to recover fetal blood and tissue has rapidly advanced this area of medicine.

Methods of prenatal diagnosis include sonography (the use of high frequency waves to record a visual image of the fetus), amniocentesis (removal and analysis of amniotic fluid surrounding the fetus), chorionic villi sampling (removal and analysis of placental tissues), and alfafetaprotein testing (screening maternal blood for elevated levels of a fetal protein which indicate a risk of neural tube defects) (Rauch, 1988).

Less common but equally important are the methods of fetal treatment, which include: surgical treatment of obstructions inutero, use of medications to treat the fetus inutero, and fetal blood transfusions (Manning, 1989).

The emotional issues for parents who choose prenatal testing and/or subsequent treatment are as follows: anxiety related to anticipating the test, tension while awaiting the test results, anxiety and guilt regarding possible side effects of the test, fear the test will reveal a problem and decision-making regarding pregnancy termination or treatment of any identified problems (Rice & Doherty, 1982; Robinson et al., 1975).

If treatment is available, parents must choose whether or not to continue with the pregnancy. These parents will confront difficult decisions about risks, anxiety related to outcomes, financial concerns and the difficulty of balancing hope and reality as they look forward to the baby's birth. Some families may decide against the treatment, and opt for continuation or termination of the pregnancy. If no treatment is available and the parents decide to continue with the pregnancy they must begin to accept the reality of the baby's anomaly and prepare themselves and their families for the birth. Sometimes families opt not to continue with the pregnancy. These parents usually require much nonjudgmental emotional support to help them to cope with such a decision.

Other Medical Problems

There are a number of medical problems and diseases that occur prior to or during pregnancy which can complicate pregnancy, and threaten the health of the mother and the fetus. Such medical problems can affect nearly all systems of the body and include chronic as well as acute complications. These problems must be monitored closely and may necessitate hospitalization and possibly surgery during pregnancy. Conditions such as heart disease, blood disorders, lung disease, arthritis, or any surgical procedure performed during pregnancy may place the mother and baby at risk (Pilliteri, 1992; Resnick & Moore, 1995).

COMMON EMOTIONAL ISSUES AMONG PERINATAL PATIENTS

In addition to the medical problems described, there are several common emotional reactions which perinatal patients seem to experience. Not all patients experience these feelings and they may be seen in varying degrees in those who do experience them. The type of medical problem, the support system available to the family, and other psychosocial factors seem to affect the type and degree of severity of these emotional reactions.

Loss of Control

As mentioned earlier, normal pregnancy is marked by intense somatic and emotional changes which in turn may result in maternal feelings of helplessness and loss of control. Bodily changes are so rampant and dramatic that mothers-to-be often report feeling as if their bodies are no longer their own. It is not surprising then that issues of control are common among the high risk population.

Complete or partial bedrest, the use of powerful tocolytics, daily insulin injections, frequent medical appointments and long or frequent hospitalizations may exacerbate the feelings of loss of control and helplessness felt by most pregnant women.

Anxiety

Most perinatal patients report feeling worried or anxious. The anxiety is often related to the uncertainty of the outcome of the pregnancy and treatment or the need for frequent visits to the clinic and/or prolonged hospitalization. These long hospital stays, marked by absence from friends or community supports, are anxiety producing for most patients. This is particularly true for patients who are hospitalized outside their communities. These patients may feel especially isolated, and require additional support to adjust to the hospital routine. For many women, hospitalization means a separation from their other children. Further, role confusion resulting from the abrupt change from caregiver to dependent recipient of care may be a source of anxiety for some. There are some parents who opt to leave the hospital against medical advice because they cannot tolerate the separation from their children and/or do not have anyone else to care for the children while they are hospitalized.

Grief

Often perinatal patients report feelings of grief or mourning related to the loss of a healthy, normal pregnancy. Though this is normal for patients who have experienced complications during pregnancy, it may be a very painful reaction often accompanied by feelings of anger, sorrow and guilt (Solnit & Stark, 1961).

Boredom

As previously mentioned, many perinatal patients must be confined to total bedrest either at home or in the hospital. For individuals who are usually very active in their work at home or in the community, this forced sedentary period can lead to boredom and frustration. The resultant feelings of resentment and anger may be, in turn, directed towards the baby. Though considered normal by most, these feelings may be a source of shame to the mother. If she is unable to express them in a supportive atmosphere, they may lead to further conflict which may present as non-compliance with medical recommendations or other acting out behaviors.

Fear

Most if not all perinatal patients report feeling fear and worry related to their baby's survival, health and well-being. Many also fear that they themselves will die or not return to their prior level of functioning. In addition, the fear their future ability to reproduce will be negatively affected by the current perinatal problem is common. Realistic reassurance, strong family and staff support, autonomy in decision making regarding treatment and privacy in which to express all concerns will help to comfort the fearful family.

Ambivalence

The experience of a high risk pregnancy often elicits feelings of ambivalence in the perinatal patient and her family. On one hand she may endure intense discomfort in order to postpone her baby's birth but at the same time may be wishing for an early delivery and an end to her ordeal. Further, she may long to be discharged home but postpone leaving the hospital for fear she will be unable to return in time for a safe controlled delivery. Often, she loves her unborn child but resents the problems associated with the pregnancy. Such feelings of intense ambivalence may be a source of confusion and guilt to the mother and reassurance that they are normal is often helpful.

Guilt

Many perinatal patients express feelings of guilt related to their own and the fetus' medical complications. Frequently, mothers on the perinatal unit will review their actions over and over again in an attempt to identify a particular event which may have precipitated the hospitalization. Whether or not the mother's behavior precipitated the medical problem, the feelings of guilt are real, and can have a strong impact on how the mother perceives herself as a parent. It is also common for one parent to blame the other for the medical complication. When this occurs, parents should be given support and realistic reassurances.

ROLE OF SOCIAL WORKER ON THE PERINATAL UNIT

The social work role on the Perinatal unit is multifaceted (Walther, 1990). It may be broadly defined as including direct services to families, work with the system and worker self care. The direct services role is made up of assessment and treatment planning, intervention and discharge planning and follow-up. The systems role involves coordination with and support of staff and teaching. Finally, the care for self has two components, peer support and self care. We begin with direct services.

Assessment

Social work services to perinatal patients and their families usually begin with assessment. The initial assessment, based on observation of the family and available social and medical history, is very important as it provides immediate support to the family which is usually in crisis. This initial contact creates a link that will enable the care team to begin to understand the family, their strengths and coping style. The early assessment also provides a foundation of trust and support on which the ongoing assessment and intervention may be built.

Following the initial crisis period and early assessment, the social worker begins to focus on more in-depth data collection including a psychosocial history and assessment of the family's emotional and cognitive response to the event. Core components of the psychosocial history include a general history of the family, a discussion of specific problems and stresses identified by the family, the patient's and/or family's prior experience with infertility, pregnancy, illness, hospitalization and loss, and an evaluation of the family's resources. The resources may include friends, family members, and social or community groups, religious beliefs and/or affiliations, health coverage, financial resources, child care, housing, transportation and general mental health (Carlton, 1984).

In-depth assessment of the family's emotional-cognitive status includes an assessment of the following factors: (1) the patient's and/or family's perceptions of the problem which led to the hospitalization, (2) the patient and/or family's understanding of what is happening to the patient, (3) the mother's and/or family's ability to adjust to the hospitalization and (4) the patient's and/or family's feelings and perceptions regarding the pregnancy (what the pregnancy means to the family).

The ongoing assessment of the family should include contact with siblings, but the other children in the system are usually absent from the medical setting. Nevertheless, their reactions to maternal separation, family disruption and the addition and/or loss of a family member need to be evaluated. Often these evaluations must be done through the parents if distance, lack of family resources, or hospital policy prevents the child from visiting the hospital. Secondhand evaluations are difficult because some parents may, in an attempt to deny their own feelings, minimize the reactions of their children. They often state that a child is too young to know what is happening or too busy to care.

Those who have studied children's reactions to perinatal events have found that even the very youngest children are affected by losses occurring during this period (Cain et al., 1964; Cavenar et al., 1979; Furlong Lind & Beck Black, 1984). Thus the social worker may intervene by helping parents recognize those feelings and help their children express them constructively.

This may be done in several ways. If parental separation is an issue, visiting should be arranged. If hospital policy is an impediment to this, the social worker should work to change it. If parental resistance is an issue, parents can be reassured that even if tears come at the end of the visit that disruption is better than an extended separation with no contact. In addition, video or audiotaped visits may help parents and children during long separations.

In the case of perinatal loss, parental attitudes about death, children's developmental stages, and knowledge about death and the child's wishes should all be assessed and weighed in deciding how involved the child should be. Generally, honesty seems to work best when discussing issues of loss and death with children. What they are told should be based on what they know about the pregnancy. If the children want to see the baby or attend the funeral that should be discussed in detail with the family, the child's pediatrician, mental health professionals and the child. The authors have found that if a child expresses an interest in being included in such rituals and if family support is good it should be considered.

Social Work Interventions and Treatment

Once the initial assessment is complete and the treatment plan made, the social worker focuses on implementing appropriate interventions. There are a variety of social work interventions that the perinatal social worker may utilize. Compton and Galaway (1984) describe 5 interventive social work roles to be used in facilitating problem solving for clients. These roles are: Social Broker, Enabler, Teacher, Mediator and Advocate. The following is a brief description of each role, and an example of how the perinatal social worker may act in these roles as part of the problem solving plan.

The social worker in the role of Social Broker refers clients to community resources for additional support. For example, he or she may refer a client to a marital counselor or day care hotline.

The social worker in the role of Enabler utilizes a variety of supportive interventions to help the client identify his/her strengths or resources to mobilize a problem solving plan. As an example, the perinatal social worker might encourage parents to explore communication problems and identify alternative approaches. The Enabler also helps the client to develop insight and encourages the client to discuss feelings related to medical or other problems while providing support and reassurance.

The perinatal social worker may also assist clients in the role of Teacher. For example, the Teacher provides clients with information about community resources, informs a mother of her rights during hospitalization, helps educate parents about high risk infants and/or orients parents to the NICU.

The social worker in the role of Advocate assists clients by speaking on their behalf to others. For example, the social worker in this role may speak with a Public Aid worker to ensure the family receives help with transportation to the hospital.

Lastly, the perinatal social worker may assume the Mediator role to facilitate resolution of disputes between the family and third parties. Some examples of this role might include mediating with parents on issues related to custody, mediating between the parents and the state child welfare agency, or mediating a dispute between the parents and their landlord (Comptom & Galaway, 1984).

Discharge Planning and Follow-Up

As stated earlier, perinatal patients often experience ambivalence at time of discharge. The social worker plays an important role in assisting families to understand their feelings and prepare for discharge home. The social worker may link the mother and/or family with community resources to provide nonmedical support and follow-up after discharge. In addition, the social worker may need to evaluate the home situation and help families secure equipment so the mother can be cared for at home. Some examples of medical equipment prescribed for home follow-up include glucometers, infusion pumps, or contraction monitors.

After discharge, the social worker may be involved with follow-up of the patient in one of the following ways. The social worker may continue to work with the family until delivery; if discharge follows delivery and the baby is in the NICU the social worker may provide continued services there; and if discharge follows delivery of a healthy baby the social worker may remain available to the family as needed to help them process their experience. Lastly, if discharge follows a perinatal loss the social worker should ideally remain available as long as the family needs support.

Work with the Interdisciplinary Team

The social worker on the perinatal unit must be prepared to work closely with multidisciplinary team members including hospital administration, legal counsel, doctors, nurses, chaplains, respiratory therapists, laboratory technicians, secretaries and transport staff. The role of coordinator and communicator with other team members is central to the functioning of the perinatal social worker. Because the social worker does not rotate off service, is a skilled listener and observer and sees the system itself as a client, s/he is well suited to this role.

Further, the social worker provides support to other team members during times of stress by helping them to define and appropriately express their feelings and concerns about patients and their families. The social worker may also act as ethical conscience in areas of confidentiality, and patient self-determination. Finally the social worker interacts with medical staff in the role of teacher, educating them in psychosocial issues, social policy, community problems and resources and human behavior and development.

Care of Self

The perinatal social work caseload is intense. When patients with difficult pregnancies do well and the outcome is good, emotion runs high but when the outcome is bad the family and staff may be devastated. It is essential that clinicians working in such settings allow themselves time to feel and time to heal. "Time to feel" means that despite the demanding and sometimes harried nature of the setting, the social worker must allow him or herself time to share feelings and questions about difficult cases with peers. To be professionally and personally isolated from team members in such a setting may be a prescription for failure. The social worker must not allow him/herself to be seen as too strong to feel pain. "Time to heal" simply means taking time after a difficult case to process what happened. Often in a health setting the expectation is that workers must rise to the occasion and go right on to the next case. Sometimes that cannot be avoided but one must always go back to do any emotional work left undone.

The perinatal social worker must learn to take advantage of all available resources including supervision, friends, family, religion, exercise, music and hobbies in order to soothe and care for him/herself. Regular days off, vacations, and institutionally-supported continuing education are essential to the continued mental and physical health of a worker in such a setting.

While objectivity and professionalism are essential in any social work position, the life and death issues dealt with daily in the perinatal setting demand an acknowledgement of the intensity of the case material and a need for support and healing.

Accepted for Publication: 05/14/96

REFERENCES

Batterman, R. (1985). A comprehensive approach to treating infertility. *Health & Social Work*, 10, 46-54.

Benson, R.C. (1986). Preterm Labor. In D.H. Danforth & J.R. Scott (Eds.), *Obstetrics & Gynecology*. Philadelphia: JB Lippincott Company, 682-689.

Berger, C.S., Sorenson, L., Gendler, B., & Fitzsimmons, J. (1990). Cocaine and pregnancy: A challenge for health care providers. *Health & Social Work*, 15 (4), 310-316.

Berkowitz, R.L. & Lynch, L. (1990). Selective reduction: An unfortunate misnomer. *Obstetrics & Gynecology*, 75, 873-874.

Bibring, G. (1959). Some considerations of the psychological processes in pregnancy. *Psychoanalytic Study of the Child*, 14, 113-121.

Bibring, G.L., Dwyer, T.F., Huntington, D.S., & Valentstein, A.F. (1961). A study of the psychological process in pregnancy and of the earliest mother-child relationship. *Psychoanalytic Study of the Child*, 16, 9-24.

Buchanan, T.A. & Couston, D.R. (1995). Diabetes mellitus. In G.N. Burrow & T.F. Ferris (Eds.), *Medical Complications During Pregnancy* (4th ed.). Philadelphia: W.B. Saunders Company, 29-54.

Cain, A.C., Erickson, M.E., Fast, I., & Vaughan, R.A. (1964). Children's disturbed reactions to their mother's miscarriage. *Psychosomatic Medicine*, 26 (1), 58-66.

Carlton, T.O. (1984). *Clinical Social Work in Health Settings*. New York: Springer Publishing Co., Chapter 4.

Cavenar, J.O., Spaulding, J.G., & Sullivan, J.L. (1979). Child's reaction to mother's abortion: Case report. *Military Medicine*, 144, 412-413.

Comptom, B. & Galaway, B. (1984). *Social Work Processes*, Third Ed. Homewood, Illinois: Dorsey Press.

Connon, J. (1995). Gastrointestinal complications. In G.N. Burrow & T.F. Ferris (Eds.), *Medical Complications During Pregnancy* (4th edition). Philadelphia: W.B. Saunders Company, 285-306.

Furlong (Lind), R.M. & Beck Black, R. (1984). Pregnancy termination for genetic indications: The impact on families. *Social Work in Health Care*, 10 (1), 17-33.

Furlong Lind, R. & Beck Black, R. (1988). Psychosocial implications, family planning & emotional support. In E.A. Reece & D.R. Coustan (Eds.), *Diabetes Mellitus in Pregnancy, Principles and Practice*. New York: Churchill Livingston, 587-598.

Giacoia, G.P. (1990). Cocaine in the cradle: A hidden epidemic. *Southern Medical Journal*, 83 (8), 947-951.

Greenfeld, D.A., Diamond, M.P., & DeCherney, A.H. (1988). Grief reactions following in-vitro fertilization treatment. *Journal of Psychosomatic Obstetrics & Gynecology*, 8, 169-174.

Harrison, Helen. (1983). *The Premature Baby Book: A Parent's Guide to Coping & Caring in the First Years*. New York: St. Martin's Press.

Johnson, J. & Daikoku, N. (1985). Prepartal rupture of the chorioamnion. In Bruce K. Young (Ed.), *The Patient Within the Patient: Problems in Perinatal Medicine*. March of Dimes Birth Defects Foundation, Birth Defects: Original Article Series, 21 (5), New York: Alan R. Liss, Inc., 73-89.

Killam, A. & Trofatter, K.F. (1986). Multiple pregnancy. In D.N. Danforth & J.R. Scott (Eds.), *Obstetrics & Gynecology*. Philadelphia: J.B. Lippincott Company, 473-480.

Kitzmiller, J.L., Cloherty, J.P., & Graham, C.A. (1982). Management of diabetes &

pregnancy. In G.P. Kozak (Ed.), *Clinical Diabetes Mellitus*. Philadelphia: W.B. Saunders Company, 203-214.

Manginello, F.P. & DiGeronimo, T.F. (1991). *Your Premature Baby*. New York: John Wiley & Sons Inc., 7-12.

Manning, F.A. (1989). General principles & application of ultrasound. In R.K. Creasy and R. Resnik (Eds.), *Maternal-Fetal Medicine: Principles & Practice*. Philadelphia: W.B. Saunders Company, 777-823.

Naeye, R.L. & Tafari, N. (1983). *Risk Factors in Pregnancy & Diseases of the Fetus & Newborn*. Baltimore: Williams & Wilkins, 145-171.

Parad, H.J. (1965). *Crisis Intervention: Selected Readings*. New York: Family Service Association of America.

Pilliteri, A. (1992). *Maternal & Child Nursing: Care of the Childbearing and Childrearing Family* (2nd Ed.). Philadelphia: J.B. Lippincott Company.

Rauch, J.B. (1988). Social work and the genetics revolution: Genetic services. *Social Work*, 33, Sept.-Oct., 389-395.

Resnick, R. & Moore, T.R. (1995). Obstetric management of the high risk patient. In G.N. Burrow & T.F. Ferris (Eds.), *Medical Complications During Pregnancy* (4th ed.). Philadelphia: W.B. Saunders Company, 285-306.

Rice, N. & Doherty, R. (1982). Reflections on prenatal diagnosis: The consumers' views. *Social Work in Health Care*, 8 (1), 47-57.

Roberts, J.M. (1989). Pregnancy-related hypertension. In R.K. Creasy & R. Resnik (Eds.), *Maternal-Fetal Medicine, Principles & Practice*. Philadelphia: W.B. Saunders Company, 777-823.

Robinson, J., Tennes, K., & Robinson, A. (1975). Amniocentesis: Its impact on mothers and infants. A 1-Year follow up study. *Clinical Genetics*, 8 (12), 97-106.

Schreiner-Engel, P., Walther, V.N., Mindes, J., Lynch, L., & Berkowitz, R. (1995). First trimester multifetal pregnancy reduction: Acute and persistent psychologic reactions. *American Journal of Obstetrics & Gynecology*, 172 (2,1), 541-547.

Shapiro, C.H. (1986). Is pregnancy after infertility a dubious joy? *Social Casework*, 66, 306-313.

Shields, D. (1974). Psychology of childbirth. *Canadian Nurse*, 70 (11), 24-26.

Solnit, A.J. & Stark, M.H. (1961). Mourning and the birth of a defective child. *Psychoanalytic Study of the Child*, 16, 523-538.

Walther, V.N. (1990). Emerging roles of social work in perinatal services. *Social Work in Health Care*, 15 (2), 35-48.

Worley, R.J. (1986). Pregnancy induced health. In D.H. Danforth & J.R. Scott (Eds.), *Obstetrics & Gynecology*. Philadelphia: J.B. Lippincott Company, 446-466.

Perinatal Social Work and the Family of the Newborn Intensive Care Infant

Debra Honig Bachman, MSW, LCSW
Regina Furlong Lind, MSW, LCSW

SUMMARY. The birth of a premature and/or sick infant challenges even the most stable, intact families. If the baby is admitted to the Newborn Intensive Care Unit (NICU), the family is further challenged by the environment in which the infant is being treated.

This article examines the most frequent causes for admission to NICU, common family reactions to such a birth and admission, social work assessment and intervention used in work with families of such patients. *[Article copies available for a fee from The Haworth Document Delivery Service: 1-800-342-9678. E-mail address: getinfo@haworth.com]*

THE BIRTH OF A PREMATURE OR SICK NEONATE

The birth of a premature and/or sick infant and the admission of the neonate to the Newborn Intensive Care Unit (NICU) is an event which stresses most families to the limit of their ability to cope.

Several authors (Breslin, 1982; Grant, 1978; Kaplan & Mason, 1965)

The authors wish to acknowledge the work of Ms. Rebecca Pruitt whose invaluable guidance, encouragement, and support played a major role in developing the original format of this project. Without her dynamic teaching and solid knowledge base of perinatal social work, this project would not have been possible.

[Haworth co-indexing entry note]: "Perinatal Social Work and the Family of the Newborn Intensive Care Infant." Bachman, Debra Honig, and Regina Furlong Lind. Co-published simultaneously in *Social Work in Health Care* (The Haworth Press, Inc.) Vol. 24, No. 3/4, 1997, pp. 21-37; and: *Fundamentals of Perinatal Social Work: A Guide for Clinical Practice with Women, Infants, and Families* (ed: Regina Furlong Lind, and Debra Honig Bachman) The Haworth Press, Inc., 1997, pp. 21-37. Single or multiple copies of this article are available for a fee from The Haworth Document Delivery Service [1-800-342-9678, 9:00 a.m. - 5:00 p.m. (EST). E-mail address: getinfo@haworth.com].

have described the family response to this experience and suggested interventions to strengthen coping. When Kaplan and Mason (1965) compared the experiences of mothers of normal, full term babies with those of mothers of prematures, they found several differences. First, the mothers of premature babies reported a feeling of shock related to the birth. The authors noted that most women do not worry about early delivery and thus are taken completely by surprise if it occurs. Secondly, mothers experiencing a normal delivery do not show an increase in tension related to the health of the baby, while mothers of prematures exhibit a heightened concern for the baby's well-being after delivery. Third, mothers of prematures are anxious about separation from the baby after delivery and at the time of discharge while mothers with normal deliveries do not have this added stress (Kaplan & Mason, 1965).

In addition to the added stress felt by the families of prematures and/or sick neonates, several authors have described psychological and developmental tasks NICU parents must master to allow healthy parent-infant attachment to develop (Breslin, 1982; Grant, 1978; Kaplan & Mason, 1965). For the purposes of this discussion, the ideas and themes of these authors will be synthesized into three general phases.

The first phase is what will be referred to as the Entry Phase. During the Entry Phase, the parents are experiencing the initial impact of the crisis and are faced with the baby's premature birth or illness and its admission to the high risk nursery. At this time they are also confronted with the critical nature of their child's condition. Usual methods of coping are tried with or without success and anxiety increases. The tasks of this first phase include learning to acknowledge and cope with this unanticipated event, grieving the loss of the wished for child, facing the potential loss of the actual child and learning to adapt to the NICU milieu.

The second phase may be referred to as the Connecting Phase because it is during this phase that new coping mechanisms are being implemented to deal with the trauma, and the parents are somewhat more at ease with the situation. The parental tasks in this phase are the continued adjustment to the NICU, development of an understanding of the realistic medical needs and status of their child, the initiation of the process of relating to their child as caregivers and assumption of the direct care of the child.

The final phase may be referred to as the Launching Phase, since it is during this period that parents begin to see the child less as a sick neonate and more as a normal baby. Parental tasks may include becoming increasingly and actively involved in the child's care, taking a more active role in decision-making regarding the child and beginning to focus on the post-hospital care of the child. Some parents may need to begin the task of learning to cope with the child's long-term disabilities, or mourning the death or dying of the infant.

It may be theorized that if parents are able to successfully complete the tasks and move from one phase to the next, then they will probably be able to begin to resolve the crisis and develop a realistic relationship with the baby.

COMMON NICU MEDICAL PROBLEMS

Many, though not all, of the neonates in the NICU are admitted for problems related to prematurity. Infants with surgical problems, congenital anomalies, genetic anomalies and birth-related complications are also seen in the NICU. A partial list of the most common medical and surgical problems of infants in the NICU follows.

Respiratory Distress Syndrome/Hyaline Membrane Disease (RDS)

This condition, often called RDS, is characterized by the lack of surfactant in the infants' lungs. Surfactant reduces tension in the air sacs, and allows expansion and inflation of the lungs (Manginello & DiGeronimo, 1991; Harrison, 1983; Moya & Clark, 1992; Pilliteri, 1992). In its absence, the lungs do not expand and inflate and oxygen is not delivered to the body as needed (Pilliteri, 1992). It is a common practice to treat RDS with supplemental surfactant. RDS is most common among neonates born before the 35th week of gestation, as prior to that surfactant has not been produced (Harrison, 1983; Moya & Clark, 1992; Pilliteri, 1992).

At some hospitals, infants with RDS are treated with oxygen which may be piped directly into a plastic tent or hood covering the baby in the isolette, or used with a ventilator (also called a respirator) which provides mechanical breathing for the highly compromised child. This is accomplished by intubating and ventilating the neonate. The ventilator will mechanically inhale and exhale for the neonate, and the amount of oxygen in the infant's blood is monitored. This is referred to as monitoring of blood gases (Moya & Clark, 1992; Pilliteri, 1992).

Slowly, carefully and continually, efforts are made to wean the infant off mechanical ventilation by gradually decreasing the amount of oxygen and the pressures used to deliver it. Early weaning is considered important as prolonged use of a ventilator can result in complications for the baby. Bronchiopulmonary Dysplasia (BPD) is such a complication. BPD is a respiratory condition involving extensive lung tissue scarring and resultant airway obstruction that requires supplemental oxygen, perhaps indefinitely (Goldberg et al., 1987; McCarthy, 1986; Moya & Clark, 1992).

Retinopathy of Prematuring

Retinopathy of Prematurity (or ROP) is a medical complication affecting one-third of all premature infants. It is an eye disease which results when developing blood vessels supplying the optic nerve are adversely affected by exposure to oxygen in the air or supplemental oxygen therapy.

It was originally believed that oxygen therapy for respiratory problems associated with prematurity caused ROP, but now it is believed that the increased oxygen the baby breathes in room air is enough to damage the developing retinal blood vessels (Manginello & DiGeronimo, 1991). This increase in oxygen contributes to development of extensive scar tissue which may lead to visual impairments, tearing and/or detachment of the retina, and possibly blindness (Harrison, 1983; Kovalesky, 1984; Pilliteri, 1992).

Intraventricular Hemorrhage (IVH)

Intraventricular Hemorrhage "is a medical condition that results from abnormal bleeding on the surface of the brain, in the substance of the brain or in the brain's central chambers that are continuous with the canal of the spinal cord" (Manginello, 1991). Bleeding usually occurs during the first few days of life. For those infants born at less than 34 weeks gestational age and/or weigh less than 3 pounds 5 ounces, IVH is almost an unavoidable consequence of prematurity (Manginello, 1991). These bleeds are graded 1 through 4. Grades 1 or 2 indicate that the bleeding will most likely resolve on its own, and are usually not associated with long-term deficits. Grades 3 or 4 indicate a more serious degree of bleeding and are more highly associated with later learning disabilities, hearing or vision deficits, Cerebral Palsy, or Hydrocephalus (excess fluid around the brain which causes pressure on tissues and can result in tissue loss). In a grade 3 or 4 bleed, blood may enter the brain tissue itself (Harrison, 1983). Finally, it should be stated that some children with IVH develop normally despite the potential seriousness of this problem.

Patent Ductus Arteriosus (PDA)

PDA is a common cardiac problem among prematures characterized by an opening in the blood vessel connecting the aorta, the main artery in the body, and the pulmonary artery, which delivers blood to the lungs. In full term babies this opening usually closes several hours after birth, but often in prematures does not close on its own. This failure of the PDA to close may result in several problems including heart murmurs, and an inability to wean quickly from the ventilator. Treatment includes use of a drug called indomethacin or, if this is unsuccessful, surgical ligation of the opening. Though this is not a major surgery, it puts the infant at risk for developing infection and recovery from surgery is an added burden to a tiny neonate. However, there are usually no complications following this surgery (Harrison, 1983; Manginello & DiGeronimo, 1991; Pilliteri, 1992).

Nutrition or Inability to Feed

Feeding and the delivery of nutrition are essential for premature babies to begin to grow (Pilliteri, 1992). Premature babies are fed slowly and in small amounts. Since many premature infants cannot suck or swallow (this occurs at 34 weeks or so) they may be fed initially with hyperalimentation lines, or nasogastric (NG) tubes (tubes placed through the nose and down to the stomach used to deliver nutrition) (Harrison, 1983; Pilliteri, 1992). Premature neonates are usually fed first through intravenous techniques, and gradually progress to NG feedings. NG feedings begin with glucose solution in neonates less than 34 weeks gestation. Otherwise, the mother's breast milk may be fed to the babies through the tubes (Harrison, 1983; Moya & Clark, 1992; Pilliteri, 1992).

Necrotizing Enterocolitis (NEC)

NEC is characterized by an inflammation of the intestine which interferes with digestion. NEC is thought to be due to poor blood flow to affected areas of the bowel. NICU babies at risk to develop NEC are those who have suffered hypoxic events and/or have had complications which may have left them in a compromised condition or as a result of infection. Since severe inflammation may lead to perforation of the intestine and spread the infection throughout the body, surgical removal of severely inflamed areas of the intestine is sometimes indicated (Harrison, 1983; Pilliteri, 1992; Moya & Clark, 1992). NEC is diagnosed by x-ray and/or by blood in the stool, and is accompanied by frequent vomiting, apnea and distended abdomen. Babies with NEC are often taken off oral feedings and fed by NG tube for several days or weeks (Moya & Clark, 1992). This can delay discharge for a substantial period of time.

Sepsis

Sepsis is a complication of prematurity in which bacteria are present in the bloodstream. The bacteria are spread to all parts of the body by the blood.

The infection is casually diagnosed by blood test or culture after changes in the infant's status are noted by the parents or staff. These changes may be subtle or devastating depending on how pervasive the infection is.

Treatments through IV or injection of antibiotics and stabilization of the baby's vital signs are usually successful. Occasionally, the infection is so overwhelming that the baby does not survive (Manginello & DiGeronimo, 1991).

COMMON EMOTIONAL ISSUES AMONG FAMILIES OF NICU PATIENTS

The emotional experiences of families in the NICU can vary greatly, though there seem to be some feelings which are shared. The following is a discussion of some of these feelings but the reader is reminded that not all of these feelings will be experienced by all families with babies in the NICU.

Guilt

Many NICU parents report feelings of guilt and responsibility for the child's medical problems. Some try to pinpoint what, if any, specific activities may have precipitated the premature delivery or the child's medical condition. Though families usually are not to blame for the neonate's condition, there are situations in which they have contributed to the child's problems, as is the case of medical sequelae following parental drug or alcohol abuse. Families should be given only realistic reassurances about their guilty feelings, and encouraged to discuss their concerns. The issue of resolution of feelings of guilt is important to address with families in order to facilitate their cognitive mastery of the crisis and allow them to care for the child.

Fear

Most families of babies in the NICU report feelings of fear usually directly related to uncertainty about the neonate's survival. These fears are varied and may change over the course of the hospitalization. Initially many family members fear that they will not be strong enough to go into the unit and hold the child. They are often reluctant to talk to the staff, fearful that the whole truth about the seriousness of the child's condition will overwhelm them. Some are concerned about the financial burden of having a child in NICU and a timely discussion with a hospital financial counselor is often appropriate.

As the discharge date approaches, parents begin to question their ability to care for the baby outside of the hospital. They fear, and sometimes quite realistically, that the baby will relapse and be re-admitted. These concerns are normal and most families are comforted somewhat by knowing they are universal.

Anxiety

In addition to fear and guilt many NICU families report feeling anxious. The most common source of anxiety is probably the uncertainty surrounding the baby's survival or long-term health and development. Parents also often express anxiety related to their ability to care for the baby, fear that they will harm the baby, and they report being worried that the staff will fail to adequately care for the baby in the event of an emergency. They also report being reluctant to express any complaint about care to the staff for fear of retribution in the form of negligence of the baby.

Helplessness

Many NICU families report feeling out of control or helpless. These feelings are probably related to several factors. First, most feel a strong need to protect and care for their infants but the NICU environment and the baby's condition often limit the contact they have with the infant, thus frustrating this fulfillment of this need.

Second, the environment may be very alienating to families. Machines, alarms and the staff's homogenous attire may all be disorienting and prevent feeling at ease or in control.

Third, the complexity of the baby's medical problems and treatment may be so overwhelming that it may take days or weeks for the family to cognitively master the facts (which may be changing from moment to moment). In the meantime, strangers to the family are making life and death decisions about the child, adding to feelings of helplessness.

Grief

Feelings of guilt, mourning and loss are common among NICU families, even when the infant survives. Solnit and Stark (1961) suggest that during pregnancy, all parents imagine the perfect child. After the delivery, parents usually give up their fantasies regarding the wished for child and most attach to the real child. If the baby is premature or very ill, this process may become more complicated. The wished for and real child may be so discrepant that an actual mourning for the lost, perfect child may take place. With a premature or sick infant, this process is further complicated by the strong possibility that the real child may not survive. Thus, parents and families may be experiencing anticipatory grief even as they try to attach to the real child (Solnit & Stark, 1961).

Some may be grieving the loss of one or more of a multiple gestation while attaching to a surviving child. The acceptance of a severely compromised child may also elicit intrinsic feelings of guilt and loss in most parents.

Finally, if the neonate(s) does not survive, parents and families are often overwhelmed with feelings of loss and grief.

ROLE OF THE SOCIAL WORKER ON THE NICU

The social worker's role in the NICU is in some ways very similar to the role of the social worker in the Perinatal unit. The aspects of direct service, work with the multidisciplinary team and care of self will be examined here with emphasis on the differences in the two settings. We begin with a word about the NICU setting itself.

In the NICU the medical state of the art is utilized in the service of the smallest, most vulnerable patients. The juxtaposition of such extremes–the tiny and helpless baby and the sophisticated biomedical equipment, prompts the observer to seek a bridge between what is scientific and what is human. The social worker functions as part of that span by helping the family bypass the technology to see their baby.

Social Work Assessment

The social worker in the NICU sometimes begins his/her work with families prior to the delivery. This contact may be brief or long-term, and may be as simple as touring a family through the nursery, or as complex as helping them make decisions regarding delivery and treatment. Whatever the circumstances, assessment is begun at the first contact and continues as the worker observes and interviews the family, reads the medical record and gathers information from the medical team. The NICU assessment always includes the added dimension of observation of the family with the baby after delivery. It is at this juncture that the growing and changing relationship between family and infant can actively be observed and supported.

Because the NICU system is a more closed system than the Perinatal unit (i.e., limited access, longer average hospitalizations, rigid rules and homogenous staff attire), the assessment may be affected in several ways. First it may focus on family adjustment to the system itself, second it may be done over a somewhat longer period of time, and third, the staff may offer more input.

Staff input into the assessment may differ in the NICU and Perinatal unit as the medical staff in the NICU is trained in Pediatrics rather than Obstetrics, and Pediatric training has historically emphasized the family and its development. Further, for better or worse the staff in the NICU often sees themselves as surrogate parents and thus play a more active role in contributing to the assessment.

The Social Work Role with Siblings

It has been well documented that perinatal events impact on other children in the family (Cain et al., 1964; Cavenar et al., 1979; Furlong Lind & Beck Black, 1988). Therefore, siblings of NICU patients should be included in the family assessment and treatment to help promote integration of the new infant into the entire family system. The birth of a premature or sick neonate and admission to the NICU create some additional dimensions for siblings which will be discussed later.

Though the siblings of NICU infants may be informed of the birth of the new baby, inability to see or touch the baby, prolonged hospitalization and limited visitation may create feelings of confusion, anxiety, disappointment, guilt and fear. In addition, extended maternal hospitalization, drastic changes in daily routine, focus of family life on hospital visitation, a feeling of tension in the home and/or demise of the neonate may increase parental separation, and family disruption intensifying their responses.

Assessment of the impact of the admission of a neonate to the NICU may be done directly with the child, or through the parents. The focus is on helping parents identify and address feelings with their children. In addition, art therapy, medical play, and use of children's books which address the birth of a sibling admitted to the NICU are interventions suggested to help parents explore and meet the emotional needs of their other children.

Social Work Intervention and Treatment

Once the assessment is complete the social worker collaborates with other team members to develop a treatment plan. The treatment plan encompasses a variety of interventions to promote healthy parent-infant attachment and encourage problem solving.

Compton and Galaway's 5 interventive roles, Social Broker, Enabler, Teacher, Mediator and Advocate, will again be considered to illustrate the services provided by the social worker in the NICU (Comptom & Galaway, 1984).

The social worker may act as Social Broker by linking families with resources in the community, for example: parent support groups for families of premature infants, electric breast pump rental companies, visiting nurses, parents of twins groups, etc. The list of possibilities may be quite extensive and the referrals will depend on the needs of the families.

There are many opportunities for the NICU social worker to act in the role of Enabler by helping families utilize their strengths to cope with the crisis of having a baby in the NICU. S/he might work intensively with the verbal, insightful family, discussing their feelings related to the ongoing NICU experience. The social worker may use this developing therapeutic relationship with the family to support parents and to promote healthy parent-infant attachment. Where appropriate, the social worker might help the family begin to focus on normal parenting behaviors such as dressing the baby, calling him/her by name, talking or singing to the baby, or putting toys or family pictures in the isolette.

The NICU social worker also helps facilitate healthy parent-infant attachment and problem solving while utilizing the Teacher role. Some examples of the NICU social worker as educator include giving parents NICU booklets which describe the unit, helping familiarize parents with the names of their baby's physicians, nurses, respiratory therapists and other members of the care team who will be involved in the care of the baby, and teaching them how to contact staff to obtain information about their baby.

The Mediator role is also an important one for the NICU social worker to use when working with parents of NICU patients. Some of the examples of this role might include mediating between the parents and the state child welfare agency, between the parents and an employer, or between parents and an insurance company (Compton & Galaway, 1984).

Lastly, the NICU social worker also helps facilitate problem solving while taking the role of the Advocate. The social worker acts as advocate by ensuring that parents know their rights to see their child, or their baby's hospital documents. When appropriate, the social worker may also help train parents to assert themselves with team members to ensure that all of their questions or concerns are addressed. Advocacy may involve assisting family and staff members in making difficult decisions regarding termination of treatment. A brief discussion of this subject will follow.

Decisions Regarding the Termination of Treatment

The guilt and devastation parents feel after the birth of a sick or premature baby may be compounded if the baby's condition is found to be incompatible with life in the absence of continued medical treatment (Breslin, 1982). At this junction the parents and staff may be confronted with the need to decide if medical interventions should continue. Most NICU's have protocols for deciding the care of such critically ill babies which they developed after the Baby Doe dilemmas of the 1980s.

Ethics Committees, consultation, informal discussion and formal patient care conferences are utilized in developing a plan. The social worker who is often already involved with the family (and may have even initiated the discussion at the parents' request) may be called upon to contribute to the decision-making process. The social worker may help families clarify and state their beliefs and wishes regarding the continuation or termination of treatment of their neonate. The social worker may also help facilitate this decision-making process by identifying and sharing information about family and community available to support whatever decision is made.

If the decision is made to terminate treatment, unit protocols should be followed to carry out a clearly agreed upon plan. (In the absence of such unit protocols please refer to Breslin's Nine Step Plan, Breslin, 1982.) Follow-up should include telephone contact and a face-to-face meeting with the parents to report autopsy results to review the details of the baby's treatment course and death, and to assess and support parental grieving (Breslin, 1982 Ch. 6).

Child Protective Cases in the NICU

In order to provide comprehensive child welfare services throughout the U.S., each state funds and operates its own child welfare agency. While the name of this agency varies from state to state, the common purpose is to provide services to ensure the welfare of children and their families. Services offered include general social services, foster care, assistance to unwed mothers, and adoption services. Suspected child abuse or neglect cases are also serviced by this agency.

All hospitals, physicians, nurses, social workers, or other medical personnel are required by law to report suspicion of abuse or neglect to the state's child welfare agency to provide a thorough investigation of the report. Based on their investigation, the state agency may either unfound the report, recommend the child remain in the home and the family receive intensive social services, or refer the case to court to take protective custody and place the child outside the home.

The NICU social worker may refer families to the state's child welfare agency for a variety of reasons including evaluation of families of infants born with Fetal Alcohol Syndrome, drug withdrawal, or maternal/fetal positive urine drug screen, prior history of or suspicion of abuse or neglect, or adoption of hard to place or abandoned infants.

Referrals may also be made for services to families with high risk social situations which may come to the attention of the social worker and staff while the baby is in the nursery. For example, parental lack of attachment to the infant, failure to visit the baby while in the hospital, and/or persistent inability to understand the baby's medical needs and prepare to meet them post discharge.

Medical testing, general social work assessment, and observation and documentation of family behavior are utilized by the interdisciplinary care team to decide whether a report of suspected abuse or neglect must be made to the state child welfare agency. Whenever possible, parents should be told that a report is being made, the reason for the report, and possible outcomes of the investigation. Often a pamphlet is available to parents to explain this process. The NICU social worker may act as liaison with the state child welfare agency, hospital staff and parents to assist the family in coping with the hospitalization, investigation and discharge plans made for the baby. Assessment of home and family safety for discharge of the baby requires careful weighing of the integrity of the family and the vulnerability of the infant. State investigation and the decision to place the baby outside of the home may elicit strong parental responses such as anger, hostility or despair. If the parents act out these feelings in the NICU, atmosphere may be disrupted and communication between parents and staff may be affected.

When protective services become involved with a family whose baby is in the NICU, the perinatal social worker's interventions may be viewed as falling into the following categories: mobilizing supportive community resources to assist the family, implementing Discharge Agreements and supporting the NICU staff. A discussion of each category will follow. It should be noted that not every NICU protective service case will require all of these interventions.

The first area of social work intervention with NICU protective service cases is the use of supportive community resources. Community resources play an important role in assisting the parents in providing for the needs of their child. If parents are receptive to referrals and interventions, the social worker should mobilize community resources including substance abuse treatment programs, 0-3 early intervention programs, public home health visiting nurses and homemakers. The state child welfare agency often collaborates with the NICU social worker and the family to help facilitate referrals to these community resources.

A second area of intervention with protective service cases in the NICU is the use of Discharge Agreements. In cases where the staff has observed and documented poor family/infant interaction at the time of visits or has observed and documented lack of visitation, the social worker may work in collaboration with the primary care team to create and implement a Discharge Agreement. The Discharge Agreement is a written document which includes the specific expectations to be met by the parents in order to demonstrate they are skilled in providing safe care for the child prior to discharge home. It is important that the expectations be reasonable and achievable by the parents.

The Discharge Agreement should include consequences for non-compliance with all aspects of the plan. Since in most states it is difficult for the state child welfare agency to found a report of neglect if a baby has never left the hospital, the Discharge Agreements can be a very important tool for the NICU social worker. These agreements should be signed by the baby's parents/caregivers, physicians, nurse, social worker and other primary care team members who are involved with the baby's care. Since this process requires time (1-2 weeks), it is helpful to identify families in which such an agreement may be necessary as early as possible prior to discharge.

After the contracts are signed, twenty-four-hour visits by parents or caregivers in the hospital may be arranged. During the visit the family is solely responsible for the care of the baby. During such a stay, the caregivers "rehearse" what it will be like to care for the baby at home. The staff is available to them as needed. Such an opportunity allows the parents and staff to further assess the family's skills and abilities to care for the baby. These 24-hour visits are not done unless the patient is considered medically stable, the parents or caregivers have received adequate education in caring for the baby and have expressed comfort with performing such care.

The final intervention is that of supporting the NICU staff. Frequently NICU staff members, whether involved directly in such cases or not, will express strong emotional reactions such as anger, sadness and/or blame. They may question the discharge plan, offer themselves as foster parents and/or even treat the family inappropriately. When this occurs, the social worker may need to spend as much time helping staff members to identify and appropriately express their feelings as is spent working with the family. The staff must be helped to develop an understanding of the parents' behaviors to see them in the context of psycho/social/cultural life of the family. The NICU social worker should help staff differentiate between malicious intent to hurt the baby and poor coping or parental deficits which may have lead to the abusive or neglectful behavior. The staff must be helped to reestablish their professional objectivity in working with the family. Lastly, the NICU social worker needs to reinforce to the staff that it is the role of the medical team to help salvage and protect positive parenting skills whenever possible rather than to judge families for their differences and difficulties.

In summary, protective service cases represent some of the most complex and time-consuming cases as they involve high risk infants of multiproblem families. The difficult case material, the need for close monitoring of the family, the increased needs of the staff, the possible acting out by family and the lack of resources all add to the difficulty of these cases which have in the past few years represented a higher proportion of the NICU workers' cases.

Discharge Planning and Follow-Up

Conscientious discharge planning is critical to ensure that parents have the resources to meet the needs of their child(ren) after leaving the hospital. One team member is usually identified as the coordinator of discharge planning. Whether it is the social worker or discharge planner, that individual must accept the primary responsibility for knowing community resources and linking families with the ones appropriate to meet their needs.

The NICU social worker may act as this coordinator or share information regarding the family and community resources which will impact on the home-care plan. Discharge planning requires the social worker to utilize his/her skills in family assessment, knowledge of medical problems and their related psychosocial issues, and resources available to parents of NICU babies.

Discharge plans cannot be made with a rubber stamp, that is, they cannot be made based solely on admitting diagnosis, race, age, or socioeconomic status. Rather, unique biopsychosocial factors must be considered carefully. Input from various members of the multidisciplinary team must be integrated in order to arrange a plan to meet the specific needs of the child and the family.

The soon to be discharged infant may require various types of services which are identified by members of the NICU team. Generally speaking, the services may be grouped into three types: discharge planning needs for strictly medical problems (Example: skilled medical facility), discharge planning for development follow-up (Example: 0-3 programs, occupational or physical therapy) and discharge planning for social welfare needs (Example: state child welfare agency). One child may receive all three types of home care services.

While discharge planning resources are specific to the individual needs and may vary in local communities, there are some universal types of resources that can be used to help children who have a variety of special health care needs.

Follow-up with families after discharge from the NICU varies according to many factors including the families' experience in the NICU, the child's diagnosis and/or status at time of discharge, the type of hospital setting (i.e., the follow-up may be built into the program) and whether the child is transferred to a new medical facility. What may be said generally is that for most parents the experience of having a child(ren) in the NICU is very disturbing and disorienting. Most families develop strong feelings (positive or negative) for the staff with whom they work during such a stressful time. It may take some time to resolve the feelings whether they be intense anger or intense dependency and a member of the staff should be available for this work. The social worker is well trained for such tasks, is usually sensitive to these issues and is more likely to be able to follow cases longer than other staff members who have less autonomy. Follow-up cannot be indefinite, however, and referrals to appropriate supportive community resources should be made as needed.

Work with the Interdisciplinary Team

The social worker practicing in the NICU must work closely with multidisciplinary hospital team members including hospital administration, legal counsel, doctors, nurses, respiratory therapists, chaplains, laboratory technicians, secretaries and transport staff. The role of coordinator and communicator with other team members is central to the functioning of the social worker on the NICU. Because the social worker does not rotate off service, is a skilled listener and observer and sees the system itself as a client, s/he is well suited to the coordination/communication role with other staff members.

Further, the social worker provides support to other team members during times of stress by helping them to define and appropriately express their feelings and concerns about patients. The social worker may also act as ethical conscience in areas of confidentiality, and patient self-determination. Finally, the social worker helps to train the medical staff in psychosocial issues, social policy, community problems and resources and human behavior and development.

As mentioned earlier, the NICU is a somewhat closed system with permeable but rigid boundaries. In this atmosphere the staff may develop values, expectations and demands which they apply to themselves and others. The team members may become somewhat rigid in these expectations and this, coupled with aforementioned tendency to adopt parental roles toward the patients, may lead to difficulties for some parents. Staff may begin to judge parents according to their own standards of good parental behavior, compare families' love for the child to their own degree of caring or may overidentify with what they refer to as "good families."

If such a judgmental attitude exists, it clouds the staffperson's ability to contribute to the assessment or treatment of the family. The social worker will often find him/herself working intensively with staff to prevent or ameliorate such a loss of professional objectivity. If the medical and nursing supervisor is cooperative, then the job is manageable, but in nurseries where either judgmental attitudes or overidentification with families is allowed to continue unchecked, families and staff alike suffer.

Care of the Self

The closed system of the NICU with all its potential difficulties is often very nurturimg and supportive of its own in times of stress. If the system is functioning well, it will allow for the expression of grief, anger and disappointment.

The NICU worker has many patients who die, some after months of hospitalization. These losses are often abrupt and unexpected and may be devastating for a new worker if s/he is left unsupported. Thus, the social worker in the NICU is encouraged to join the other members of the team in appropriate mourning, which may include attending funerals, organizing memorial services at the hospital or simply crying with a co-worker.

In addition to team support, the NICU social worker must learn to take advantage of all available resources including supervision, friends, family, religion, exercise, music and hobbies in order to soothe and care for him/herself. Frequent days off, vacations and institutionally supported continuing education are essential to the continued mental and physical health of a worker in such a setting.

While objectivity and professionalism are essential in any social work position, the life and death issues dealt with daily in the NICU setting demand an acknowledgement of the intensity of the case material and a need for support and healing.

Accepted for Publication: 05/14/96

REFERENCES

Breslin, R.L. (1982). Family crisis care in the newborn special care unit. In A. Milunsky, E. Friedman, & L. Gluck (Eds.), *Advances in Perinatal Medicine*. Plenum Publishing Corporation, 312-370.

Cain, A.C., Erickson, M.E., Fast, I., & Vaughan, R.A. (1964). Children's disturbed reactions to their mother's miscarriage. *Psychosomatic Medicine*, 26 (1), 58-66.

Cavenar, J.O., Spaulding, J.G., & Sullivan, J.L. (1979). Child's reaction to mother's abortion: Case report. *Military Medicine*, 144: 412-413.

Comptom, B. & Galaway, B. (1984). *Social Work Processes*, Third Ed. Homewood, Illinois: Dorsey Press.

Furlong Lind, R. & Beck Black, R. (1988). Psychosocial implications, family planning & emotional support. In E.A. Reece & D.R. Coustan (Eds.), *Diabetes Mellitus in Pregnancy, Principles and Practice*. New York: Churchill Livingston, 587-598.

Goldberg, A.I., Noah, Z., Fleming, M., Stainek, L., Childs, B., Frost, L., & Glyn, W. (1987). Quality of care for children who require prolonged ventilation. *Quality Review Bulletin*, 13 (3), 81-88.

Grant, P. (1978). Psychosocial needs of families of high risk infants. *Family & Community Health*, 1: 91-102.

Harrison, Helen. (1983). *The Premature Baby Book: A Parent's Guide to Coping & Caring in the First Years*. New York: St. Martin's Press.

Kaplan, D.M. & Mason, E.A. (1965). Maternal reactions to premature birth viewed as an acute emotional disorder. In H.J. Parad (Ed.), *Crisis Intervention: Selected Readings*. New York: Family Service Association of America, 118-128.

Kovalesky, A. (1984). *Nurses' Guide to Children's Eyes*. New York: Grune & Stratton, Inc., 143-147.

Manginello, F.P. & DiGeronimo, T.F. (1991). *Your Premature Baby*. New York: John Wiley & Sons, Inc., 280.

McCarthy, M.F. (1986). A home discharge program for ventilator assisted children. *Pediatric Nursing*, 12 (5), 331-335, 380.

Moya, F.R. & Clark, D.A. (1992). Common problems of the newborn. In E.A. Reece, J.C. Hobbins, M.J. Mahoney, & R.H. Petrie (Eds.), *Medicine of the Fetus & Mother*. Philadelphia: J.B. Lippincott Company, 1525-1553.

Pilliteri, A. (1992). *Maternal & Child Nursing: Care of the Childbearing & Childrearing Family* (2nd ed.). Philadelphia: J.B. Lippincott.

Solnit, A.J. & Stark, M.H. (1961). Mourning and the birth of a defective child. *Psychoanalytic Study of the Child*, 16: 523-538.

Infertility
and Assisted Reproductive Technology:
The Role of the Perinatal Social Worker

Dorothy A. Greenfeld, MSW, CISW

SUMMARY. The inability to conceive a pregnancy can cause disruption and anguish to individuals and couples sharing that experience. The treatments for infertility, especially those involving assisted reproductive technology such as in vitro fertilization, can be physically, financially and emotionally stressful for participants. The impact of infertility and its treatment has introduced a new venue for perinatal social worker services to counsel, educate and support these patients. *[Article copies available for a fee from The Haworth Document Delivery Service: 1-800-342-9678. E-mail address: getinfo@haworth.com]*

INTRODUCTION

Infertility–defined as the inability to achieve pregnancy after one year of unprotected sexual intercourse–appears to be on the increase. Currently in the United States, one in six couples experiences infertility during their childbearing years. The causes of infertility and the increase in the problem are not completely understood, but appear to be a combination of sociological, medical and environmental factors. For example, couples are

Dorothy A. Greenfeld is affiliated with Yale New Haven Hospital, Department of Social Work, New Haven, CT.

[Haworth co-indexing entry note]: "Infertility and Assisted Reproductive Technology: The Role of the Perinatal Social Worker." Greenfeld, Dorothy A. Co-published simultaneously in *Social Work in Health Care* (The Haworth Press, Inc.) Vol. 24, No. 3/4, 1997, pp. 39-46; and: *Fundamentals of Perinatal Social Work: A Guide for Clinical Practice with Women, Infants, and Families* (ed: Regina Furlong Lind, and Debra Honig Bachman) The Haworth Press, Inc., 1997, pp. 39-46. Single or multiple copies of this article are available for a fee from The Haworth Document Delivery Service [1-800-342-9678, 9:00 a.m. - 5:00 p.m. (EST). E-mail address: getinfo@haworth.com].

waiting longer to start their families, and female fertility decreases with age. An increase in sexually transmitted diseases, complications from the IUD, and repeated abortions can lead to pelvic inflammatory disease which may in turn increase the rate of infertility. Finally, environmental and occupational hazards of exposure to toxins such as radiation, lead and pesticides, can contribute to infertility (Speroff, Glass and Kase, 1989).

Who are the infertile? Although infertile women are more likely to be black than white, more likely to be older rather than younger, and more likely to have less than a high school education, these are not the characteristics of the women most likely to seek treatment in the infertility clinics. Those seeking treatment are typically part of the young, white, well-educated and well-motivated "baby boom generation" who can afford treatment and who account for the increased demand for infertility services in recent years (Mueller and Daling, 1989).

Whatever their socioeconomic status, however, the experience of infertility is well documented as a source of profound sadness and stress to women and their partners who are trying unsuccessfully to have children (Valentine, 1986; Covington, 1987). In addition, the emotional demands of infertility can have a profound impact on the marital and sexual relationship of the couple. Indeed, this experience may have a significant effect on how they relate to families and friends as well. For example, couples who are having difficulty conceiving a pregnancy may decide for reasons of confidentiality to keep this problem to themselves. Although this may help them to maintain a sense of privacy in the short run, in the long run secrecy may increase their sense of isolation and/or leave them open to insensitive comments such as "so when are you going to have a family?"

It is easy to see why couples may choose to be secretive about their inability to achieve a pregnancy. Despite the fact that in recent years infertility and reproductive technology have received a great deal of media attention, leading to more openness about the subject, there nevertheless remains a stigma associated with being infertile in a very fertile world. Although pregnancy is, literally, the cure for infertility, problems during pregnancy, labor or birth can reawaken and exacerbate sensitive psychological issues associated with infertility. These issues include vulnerability, loss of self esteem, and a sense that one's body is defective (Lind, Pruitt and Greenfeld, 1990). The perinatal social worker's first introduction to this population is often when the formerly infertile woman appears in the hospital with problems in pregnancy and/or is overwhelmed by the birth of a premature or sick child. The patient's apparent "overreaction" to her situation is more clearly understood by the perinatal social worker who appreciates the psychological consequences of infertility and who has an understanding of the physical, financial, social and emotional impact of infertility.

BACKGROUND

As recently as 25 years ago, the etiology of infertility–particularly in women–was considered to be psychological. Women who had trouble conceiving were thought to be ambivalent about motherhood and to have "unresolved conflicts" with their own mothers. Clinicians of that era subscribed to the sexist stereotype of the infertile female as a narcissistic and hysterical woman who psychologically contributed to "her own infertility problem" (Deutsch, 1945). This notion continued into the 1960s, particularly among women with "unexplained infertility."

However, in recent decades a great deal has been learned about the etiology of infertility. As more information about such problems as anovulation, congenitally malformed reproductive organs, blocked fallopian tubes and endometriosis (to name but a few) became available, new and increasingly effective treatments were devised. In addition, in the 1970s, Barbara Eck Menning, a nurse who was herself infertile, began a conceptual revolution when she asserted that infertility and its treatment *caused* anxiety and stress rather than *resulted* from it. Ms. Menning formed a support group for infertile couples which ultimately led to a national support network known as RESOLVE, Incorporated, which now has branches in all fifty states. She has written several papers describing the medical aspects of infertility and its treatment and was among the first to point out that the emotional ups and downs of infertility are a *normal* response to the problem (Menning, 1980).

Although current public awareness of infertility and its treatment has advanced considerably, there remain a number of myths associated with infertility that contribute to a distorted view of infertile patients and which contribute to the discomfort and isolation experienced by infertile couples. These myths include the following: (1) infertility is a woman's disease (in fact, 50% of infertility is a male problem); (2) that if a couple adopts a child they are very likely to achieve pregnancy soon thereafter (in fact, this occurs only in about 5% of infertile couples who adopt a child); (3) that infertility is the result of a sexual problem: that is, to say that infertile women are "frigid" and infertile men are "impotent" (in fact, the problem of infertility can adversely affect the sexual functioning of an infertile couple, but infertility resulting from sexual problems is relatively rare); (4) that if a woman can get pregnant once she can always get pregnant again (in fact, secondary infertility is very common); and (5) that infertility is psychological and that if a woman could learn to "relax" properly she could become pregnant (Speroff, Glass and Kase, 1989; Menning, 1980).

INFERTILITY TREATMENT

Types of Treatment

Treatment for infertility often involves a long and physically grueling process. The work-up for infertility generally begins after a couple has failed to achieve conception after a year of unprotected sexual intercourse. The treatment regime may range from the seemingly benign daily monitoring of the woman's temperature to a more physically and emotionally complicated schedule involving "specifically timed sexual intercourse." Still more complex and invasive treatment may include surgery, ovarian stimulation with fertility hormones, and/or the use of assisted reproductive technology (ART) treatments such as in vitro fertilization (IVF).

IVF is a four-step process. The initial phase involves stimulation of the ovaries with a fertility drug which is self-administered by injection. The drug causes multiple ova to "ripen." The second phase is retrieval of the egg(s) by laparoscopy or by needle guided aspiration using vaginal ultrasound. In the third phase, any retrieved eggs are mixed with the male partner's semen in a petri dish to achieve fertilization. The cycle is completed with the fourth and final step in which the fertilized eggs (now embryos) are transferred into the woman's uterus. Having completed a cycle, there is no guarantee of pregnancy. In fact, the treatment has only a 15 to 20 percent chance of success.

There are many adjunct therapies to ART treatments that are making this technology available to an expanded population of patients. For example, infertile couples may now make use of embryo cryopreservation (where extra embryos are stored and frozen until the couple decides to use them or dispose of them), donor eggs (for women who, because of age, previous illness, or congenital problems cannot produce their own eggs), surrogacy (where another woman is artificially inseminated by the infertile woman's partner and carries the baby for the infertile couple) and gestational surrogacy (where a woman allows a fertilized ovum to be implanted in her uterus to carry the genetic baby of a woman who has no uterus).

Demands of the Treatment

Infertility treatments are expensive. For example, ART procedures cost between $4,000 and $10,000 per treatment cycle and are usually only partially covered by insurance (if at all). The physical and financial stress of the treatments often cause psychological stress for couples entering these programs. Participants describe a recurring cycle of hope and despair that is commonly referred to as the "rollercoaster" effect of infertility and its treatment. Women in particular experience this time as a constant state of limbo. They feel torn between the feeling that they cannot plan their lives properly–since they may get pregnant–and the fearful dread that they may never achieve pregnancy. During this time women describe a profound sense of emotional confusion–feelings of anger, worthlessness and hopelessness combined with a profound sense of loss. Furthermore, because these treatments involve conception outside of the body, they may present novel ethical dilemmas to patients. For example, if these therapies are not sanctioned by the patients' religion, the couple may find themselves cut off from yet another source of support: their church.

When the Treatment Fails

The experience of infertility and the failure of infertility treatment can have a long lasting psychological effect on women and their partners. If the treatment fails, individuals and couples often experience a period of discouragement and sadness that can at times be frightening in its emotional intensity. Several studies have reported that this is a normal response to a failed cycle of treatment. More unusual is the occasional severe grief reaction to a failed ART cycle (Greenfeld, Diamond and DeCherney, 1985). Despite the significance of this response, couples often choose to enter another treatment cycle, thereby starting the cycle of hope and despair over again. Their hope and determination that each oncoming cycle will be the one "that works" makes the grieving process difficult to resolve. The grieving is especially difficult because it is continuous and without any tangible product to bury and to bid farewell. A frequent complaint from infertile couples is the frustration they experience in the paradox they face: the treatment which inhibits the resolution of their grief is the very entity that may possibly provide the solution to their dilemma and resolve their grief.

One of the most difficult decisions facing these couples as well as the treatment teams is when to recommend ending treatment. For some couples this is an evolutionary process, they set their own goals and are clear about where their limits are and when to stop. However, for many, the thought of facing a childless future or considering other options is frightening, and the ever expanding treatment technology is too captivating. This has become an especially difficult question since the treatment is ever expanding and ongoing. For example, until recently even women determined to continue treatment until it was successful were eventually stopped in their quest by the reality of menopause. That is no longer the case. Donor egg programs have now made pregnancy possible for menopausal and post menopausal women.

Pregnancy after infertility: Focused as they are on their menstrual cycle, the treatment and the recurring fear of disappointment, infertility patients often find the transition from infertility to pregnancy surprisingly difficult. One way that infertile women cope with their inability to conceive is to protect themselves emotionally by avoiding becoming "too hopeful." Some treatments–particularly those that involve the use of fertility drugs– can exacerbate their hope and despair by "playing tricks" on the body. An example is what Sandelowski et al. (1990) refer to as a "drug induced pseudopsyesis"–i.e., sore breasts, nausea and a delayed menses. Thus, it is no surprise that women have doubts when they *do* become pregnant. In early pregnancy the formerly infertile patient may experience what Olshansky (1990) refers to as an "identity shift" from infertile woman to normal pregnant woman. Once the pregnancy is clearly documented the woman may enter into what Sandelowski et al. refer to as a "waiting to lose phase," meaning that she guards against the possibility of suffering another painful disappointment by preparing herself to lose the pregnancy. For some formerly infertile women this heightened sense of vulnerability can continue throughout the pregnancy and even following the baby's birth. Although this apprehension appears to be temporary and related to the long standing infertility, the experience can be complicated by a difficult pregnancy, a high risk pregnancy and/or problems with labor and birth. If, for example, the infant needs to be admitted to the Newborn Intensive Care Unit, the mother may psychologically experience the hospitalization as resulting from her "defective reproductive apparatus" even though the reason for the baby's admission may be unrelated to the mother's prior infertility. For such women the agony of infertility and the sense that "nothing her body does is okay" may be continually reawakened (Lind, Pruitt and Greenfeld, 1990).

Multifetal pregnancies: A consequence of the increase in infertility treatments–especially those that involve the use of infertility drugs and IVF–is an increased number of multifetal pregnancies. These pregnancies, especially those involving triplets and greater, often result in prematurity (Berkowitz). Patients with multifetal pregnancies are often encouraged to consider multifetal pregnancy reduction, a procedure which involves the termination of part of their pregnancy. This option is not available everywhere, so couples often have to travel great distances for a procedure which is controversial and emotionally and physically difficult.

Social Work Intervention

The social worker typically encounters these couples in the infertility treatment setting. However, there are a variety of settings in which the perinatal social worker may meet with the infertile or formerly infertile patient couples and where a grasp of the emotional impact of infertility and its treatment can be extremely helpful and comforting to these patients. By virtue of their infertility treatment, these couples are deeply involved in an arcane world of mystifying terminology and procedures and they are deeply appreciative when they find a counselor who is knowledgeable and can speak and understand that language.

The role of social work with infertile couples has been well established as one that involves education as well as support (Greenfeld, Diamond and DeCherney, 1985; Valentine, 1986; & Covington, 1987). Since infertility treatments are evolving rapidly, the social worker needs to acquire and maintain an up-to-date knowledge of the specialized area of assisted reproduction. The complicated treatment decisions and the psychological impact of these treatments, as well as the process of infertility and ongoing loss, call for social work intervention in this setting.

Common Treatment Issues

Because infertility commonly has an adverse effect on the patient's self esteem and the couple's sexual relationship, it often feels like an ongoing and debilitating crisis. Most infertile couples can benefit from counseling, either as individuals or as couples. For many, more focused intervention such as sexual therapy or bereavement counseling may be indicated.

A more general and particularly crucial role for social work is the provision of support which "normalizes" the experience of the individual or couple. Under the prolonged stress of infertility treatment, some patients have a tendency to fear that things are beyond their control and that they are "going crazy." They are typically greatly reassured when they learn that it is *normal* to feel resentful toward women who are pregnant, *normal* to want to avoid baby showers and *normal* to feel ongoing grief for something that does not exist.

One of the most effective methods available for this normalization process is to provide infertile couples with access to others just like them. To most infertile couples the world feels like a very fertile place. Therefore, they are often greatly reassured by participation in support groups for the infertile, whether professionally led or of the "self-help" variety. Resolve, Inc., a nationwide support network for infertility, provides education, support and help to couples across the country. Social workers working with this population should have information available to people about this network.

CONCLUSION

Infertility and its treatment can cause a disheartening and disruptive period in the lives of individuals and couples. Assisted reproductive technology, while offering the hope of a successful pregnancy, can be emotionally as well as financially costly. ART treatment areas have offered a whole new venue for perinatal social workers. Social workers who understand the treatment can educate, counsel and support patient couples experiencing this disruption in their lives.

Accepted for Publication: 05/15/96

REFERENCES

Berkowitz, R., Lynch, L., Chkara, U., Wilkins, I., Melialeh, K., Alvarez, E. (1988). Selective reduction of multifetal pregnancies in the first trimester. *New England Journal of Medicine* 318:16.

Covington, S.N. (1987). Psychosocial evaluation of the infertile couple: Implications for social work practice. In *Infertility and Adoption: A Guide for Social Work Practice*. New York: The Haworth Press, Inc.

Deutsch, H. (1945). *The Psychology of Women*. New York: Grune and Stratton. Vol II.

Greenfeld, D.A., Diamond, M.P., DeCherney, A.H. (1985). Grief reactions following treatment for in vitro fertilization. *Social Work in Health Care*.

Lind, R.F., Pruitt, R.L., Greenfeld, D.A. (1990). The newborn intensive care unit experience for previously infertile couples. *Health and Social Work*.

Mahlstedt, P.P. (1985). The psychological component of infertility. *Fertility and Sterility* 43:335.

Menning, B.E. (1980). The emotional needs of infertile couples. *Fertility and Sterility* 34:313.

Mueller, B.A., Daling, J.R. (1989). In M.R. Soules (Ed.), *Controversies in Reproductive Endocrinology and Infertility*. New York: Elsevier.

Olshansky, E.F. (1990). Psychosocial implication of pregnancy after infertility. *NAA COGS Clin Issu Perinat Womens Health Nurs* 3:342.

Sandelowski, M., Harris, B.G., Holdeich-David, D. (1990). Pregnant moments: The process of conception in infertile couples. *Research in Nurse & Health* 13:273.

Speroff, L., Glass, R.H., Kase, N.G. (1989). *Clinical Gynecologic Endocrinology and Infertility*. Baltimore: Williams and Wilkins.

Valentine, D.P. (1986). Psychological impact of infertility: Identifying issues and needs. *Social Work in Health Care* 11:61.

Counseling Prenatal Diagnosis Patients: The Role of the Social Worker

Patricia E. Fertel, ACSW, LISW
Rosemary E. Reiss, MD

SUMMARY. In the 1990s, new techniques and therapies for fetal problems continue to develop. Prenatal technology now provides information regarding unborn children which can sometimes be negative. This paper addresses the counseling techniques and therapeutic approaches perinatal social workers can use when dealing with parents who are confronted by hard choices regarding their pregnancies. *[Article copies available for a fee from The Haworth Document Delivery Service: 1-800-342-9678. E-mail address: getinfo@haworth.com]*

Prenatal diagnosis of fetal abnormalities has become more common and more precise over the past 15 years. The rapid development of new molecular genetic techniques has led to the identification of genes for many inherited disorders. This means that serious or progressively lethal medical conditions such as hemophilia, muscular dystrophy, cystic fibrosis, Tay-Sachs, sickle cell disease and Fragile X syndrome can be identified or ruled out in a fetus carried by a woman with a family history of these

Patricia E. Fertel is Senior Perinatal Social Worker, The Ohio State University Medical Center, College of Medicine, High Risk Perinatal Project, N118 Doan Hall, 410 West 10th Avenue, Columbus, OH 43210. Rosemary E. Reiss is Associate Professor, Obstetrics and Gynecology, Clinical Director of Prenatal Diagnosis, The Ohio State University Medical Center, Division of Maternal-Fetal Medicine, 1654 Upham Drive, 521 Means Hall, Columbus, OH 43210.

[Haworth co-indexing entry note]: "Counseling Prenatal Diagnosis Patients: The Role of the Social Worker." Fertel, Patricia E., and Rosemary E. Reiss. Co-published simultaneously in *Social Work in Health Care* (The Haworth Press, Inc.) Vol. 24, No. 3/4, 1997, pp. 47-63; and: *Fundamentals of Perinatal Social Work: A Guide for Clinical Practice with Women, Infants, and Families* (ed: Regina Furlong Lind, and Debra Honig Bachman) The Haworth Press, Inc., 1997, pp. 47-63. Single or multiple copies of this article are available for a fee from The Haworth Document Delivery Service [1-800-342-9678, 9:00 a.m. - 5:00 p.m. (EST). E-mail address: getinfo@haworth.com].

47

problems. Even women with low-risk pregnancies are now candidates for screening with maternal serum alpha-fetoprotein for anatomic defects such as spina bifida or chromosomal abnormalities such as Down syndrome. As ultrasound technology has improved and become widely available, the early diagnosis of structural birth defects has become more common.

With increased detection of congenital anomalies, more women and their families are faced with difficult choices. First, they must choose whether to avail themselves of prenatal testing. Second, if an anomaly is found, they must decide how to respond to the result. Often these decisions require integration of complex medical information and must be made within pressing time constraints. Optimally, the services of a social worker should be available to help these clients with their significant needs at this time of crisis.

Counseling is best conducted in concert with other health professionals as part of an interdisciplinary team including physicians, genetic counselors and nurses. In order to provide effective counseling, it is important for the perinatal social worker to be familiar and comfortable with the special needs of these clients and to have knowledge about:

1. the available prenatal tests
2. the types of diagnoses necessitating decision-making
3. crisis intervention
4. the grief and mourning process
5. available procedures for pregnancy termination
6. available financial and medical resources.

PRENATAL TESTING

Prenatal testing techniques include an array of options. Some do not involve any risk to the developing fetus and are offered as a screen in both low- and high-risk pregnancies. These would include ultrasound (sonogram) and maternal serum alpha-fetoprotein screening, a test on maternal blood which measures the amount of a fetal protein which crosses the placenta. A lower than normal alpha-fetoprotein (AFP) raises the patient's risk for chromosomal abnormalities. A higher than normal AFP may indicate a fetal neural tube defect or other malformation, and is an indication for further testing. Ultrasound allows visualization of the fetus and placenta to provide information about the rate of fetal growth and the presence or absence of birth defects. For example, an ultrasound could clarify whether a patient with an elevated AFP had a fetus with an anomaly or whether there was another explanation for the high value, such as twins or a more advanced gestation.

More invasive tests which sample cells derived from the fetus are only considered in pregnancies at higher risk. They may be used to make a definitive diagnosis if a screening test suggests a problem, or they may be elected by couples who know they are at risk because of age or a family history of a genetic disorder. Chorionic villus sampling (CVS) of placental tissue is usually performed between 9 and 12 weeks gestation. It involves passing a sampling device to biopsy the placental tissue under ultrasound guidance. It can be performed either transvaginally or transabdominally. After 12 weeks gestation, amniotic fluid containing fetal cells can be obtained by amniocentesis, the placement of a needle into the amniotic sac under ultrasound guidance. Fetal blood can be obtained by guiding a slender needle into the fetal umbilical cord after 18 weeks gestation in a procedure known as cordocentesis or PUBS (percutaneous umbilical blood sampling). These procedures involve a risk of miscarriage ranging from 0.3% for amniocentesis to 1% for cordocentesis. New techniques to recover fetal cells from the mother's blood without risk to the fetus are under investigation.

The samples obtained from chorionic virus sampling, amniocentesis or cordocentesis contain cells with the same genetic composition as the fetus. Tests on these cells can provide information about fetal karyotype (chromosomes), biochemical characteristics or DNA composition. In addition, alpha-fetoprotein can be measured in amniotic fluid. One to three weeks are often required from the time the samples are obtained until final results are available. Some tests, such as karyotype analysis on fetal blood, can be performed in a few days. For many families, the wait for the test results can be a very anxious period.

Case Example 1

At two months of age, the infant of a young couple is observed to have a progressive neurologic disorder. The infant is diagnosed as having Werdnig-Hoffman, a lethal autosomal recessive disease. The parents are informed that the risk of recurrence in future pregnancies is 1 in 4. The infant dies at 7 months of age. Prenatal diagnosis was not available at the time of the child's death, but a blood sample was banked to be available in the future. The couple was initially reluctant to attempt another pregnancy. Two years later DNA probes became available to enable prenatal diagnosis of Werdnig-Hoffman in this family. The couple became pregnant and elected to have chorionic villus sampling to determine whether this child was affected, unaffected or a carrier. Three weeks later, testing showed the child to be unaffected. The parents were extremely relieved and began telling friends about the pregnancy.

TYPES OF DIAGNOSES

Congenital anomalies can be classified into broad categories that also relate to methods of diagnosis and recurrence risks (see Table 1).

Karyotype abnormalities, also called aneuploidies, are abnormalities of chromosome number or shape. They form three basic groups: *trisomies*, *monosomies*, and *chromosomal rearrangements*. Normally, the cells in human tissues have 46 chromosomes: 2 of each of 22 somatic chromosomes and 2 sex chromosomes. If the egg or sperm cell which gives rise to an embryo has an extra copy of a chromosome, this leads to a *trisomy*. Trisomies are always associated with mental retardation. Trisomy 21 or Down syndrome is the most common trisomy. It occurs when there are 3 copies of chromosome 21. Most other trisomies are lethal and lead to miscarriage during the pregnancy. Some other trisomies (trisomies for chromosomes 13, 15 or 18) can lead to the birth of a live child who may also have visible structural defects and who usually dies within hours or weeks of birth. *Monosomy* occurs when only one copy of a certain chromosome is present. Monosomies are all lethal except for the monosomy of the sex chromosome where only one X is present. This karyotype is known as Turner's syndrome. Turner's is a very common cause of miscarriage, but some of these fetuses can survive to have only minor birth defects. Trisomies and monosomies occur more commonly as maternal age rises. They are not hereditary.

Chromosomal rearrangements include translocations, duplications or deletions where there is an extra or missing portion of a chromosome. Unbalanced translocation of large portions of chromosomes can produce infants with features of Down syndrome or other trisomies. They can arise as new problems or be passed down through a family. A balanced translocation is one where chromosomal material is arranged in an unusual way, but a normal amount of genetic material is present. These individuals are normal. A normal adult with a balanced translocation will have a high miscarriage rate and a 2-12% risk of an abnormal fetus or an aneuploid fetus in each ongoing pregnancy.

The second broad group of genetic disorders are *Mendelian disorders* because their inheritance follows one of the patterns described by Gregor Mendel in the 19th century. This group of disorders includes conditions such as: sickle cell disease, hemophilia, cystic fibrosis, Tay-Sachs, Marfan syndrome and muscular dystrophy. Usually these disorders result from a

TABLE 1. Congenital Disorders Amenable to Prenatal Diagnosis

TYPE	EXAMPLE	SCREENING TEST	DIAGNOSTIC TEST
Aneuploidy			
Trisomy	Down syndrome	MS-AFP, Triple screen	Karyotype
Monosomy	Turner's syndrome	Ultrasound	(CVS, amniocentesis
Triploidy			cordocentesis)
Translocation			
Mendelian			
Autosomal recessive	Cystic fibrosis	Family history, DNA analysis of parents	DNA analysis (CVS, amnio, cordo)
	Infantile polycystic kidney	Family history	Ultrasound
Autosomal dominant	Osteogenesis Imperfecta	Family history	Ultrasound
Sex-linked recessive	Duchenne's Muscular Dystrophy	Family history, DNA analysis of parents	DNA analysis (CVS, amnio, cordo)
Anatomic			
Congenital heart defects			Ultrasound
Neural tube defects	Anencephaly, Spina bifida	MS-AFP	
Abdominal wall defects	Omphalocele, gastroschisis	MS-AFP	
Many others			

mutation within a gene and may sometimes arise if a single crucial molecule of DNA is abnormal. These small DNA substitutions, deletions or duplications prevent the individual from making certain enzymes or other proteins or cause them to make faulty proteins. They are often lethal or progressively debilitating. They usually do not produce any outward physical deformities in the developing fetus which could be visible on ultrasound. For a couple with a previously affected infant, the recurrence risk ranges from 25% for autosomal recessive to 50% for autosomal dominant. Autosomal dominant disorders may also arise as new mutations. In that case, the risk of recurrence in a sibling is minimal, but risk of transmission to offspring of the affected individual is 50%, if the defect is compatible with survival.

Prenatal diagnosis using biochemical or molecular DNA techniques is available for many of these Mendelian disorders via CVS or amniocentesis. However, only families already known to be at risk are tested for them. Often, a large number of family members apart from the parents must be tested to enable prenatal diagnosis.

Anatomic or structural birth defects are abnormalities in the formation of an external or internal fetal organ. The most common structural abnormalities are neural tube defects (spina bifida and anencephaly), heart defects, defects in abdominal wall closure (omphalocele, gastroschisis), cleft lip or palate or anomalies of the gastrointestinal or urinary tract. Some of these abnormalities elevate the level of alpha-fetoprotein in the maternal blood or amniotic fluid. Most can be detected by ultrasound in the 2nd trimester. The prognosis for an infant with a structural anomaly depends on the nature of the defect and whether it is isolated or part of a syndrome of multiple defects. Structural defects are most often sporadic or multifactorial in inheritance with the precise cause difficult to identify. The recurrence risks for these range from 1-5%.

There are overlaps between these categories of fetal anomalies. Fetuses with aneuploidies have structural defects visible on ultrasound 30-50% of the time. For example, fetuses with Down syndrome sometimes have heart or gastrointestinal malformations. Mendelian syndromes occasionally produce structural defects as well. If the fetus is found to have a structural defect when ultrasound is performed, the physician will often recommend obtaining a karyotype by amniocentesis or cordocentesis to provide further information to the parents for help in their decision-making.

Case Example 2

On routine screening, a 29-year-old woman is found to have an elevated value of maternal serum alpha-fetoprotein. At 19 weeks gestation, an ultrasound shows an omphalocele, an opening of the skin of the abdomen allowing fetal bowel to protrude in a membrane covered sac. The family is counseled that this anomaly is repairable if it is an isolated problem, but that one-third of fetuses with omphaloceles also have a lethal trisomy. The family elects to have cordocentesis performed to obtain a rapid chromosomal analysis. Two days later they learn that their fetus has a normal female karyotype. Their physician arranges for them to discuss the likelihood of a successful repair with a pediatric surgeon. The family does this, and decides to continue the pregnancy. The perinatal social worker meets with them to explore their feelings, assess their circumstances and arranges for them to tour the intensive care nursery in advance of their baby's delivery.

CRISIS INTERVENTION

When a family consults a physician for prenatal diagnosis, they may or may not be expecting that something is amiss with their pregnancy. At the moment when an unfavorable diagnosis is confirmed, the patient and family are in a psychological state of shock as they plunge into crisis. The role of the social worker who meets the family at this time is to help them begin to deal with the information given them, assess some strengths, mobilize some support and promote their grieving process. The following material will describe social work practice with these special patients and their families and will include some illustrative case examples.

A THEORETICAL APPROACH
FOR PRENATAL DIAGNOSIS COUNSELING

Families who are facing uncertain pregnancy outcomes have many needs which have been summarized by Van Putte.[1] These include:

- communication in understandable terms
- reinforcement of diagnosis (education and information about the fetal problem)
- nondirective support for decision-making
- information regarding termination procedures and risks, and
- validation of worth and assistance in dealing with lowered self-esteem.

COMMUNICATION IN UNDERSTANDABLE TERMS

Dealing with families who are in crisis and mourning can be a daunting prospect for a social worker. However, being aware of common reactions and some advance preparation can allay some fears and can give the social worker more control. If possible, reading the chart, talking to another health professional who has already met the patient and gathering written materials facilitates the interviewing process.

Entering the room and beginning the interview can be difficult. Nonverbal communication can set the stage for the family's comfort level. Sitting down, drawing a chair close to the patient and providing tissues lets the family know they have your full attention and consideration. A good opening is an acknowledgment of the situation and the family's grief. For example: "Hello, my name is_____. Dr Smith has told me about your baby's problem and I'm so sorry. Can you tell me what you know about your baby?"

The patient/family will likely respond to the question and the social worker can begin to assess the patient/family's awareness of the seriousness of the problem and her/their reaction to this news. Reactions to learning a poor prognosis for the pregnancy vary widely based on a myriad of variables but usually reflect one of the stages of grief and mourning, such as: shock, denial, sadness or anger. If the diagnosis is new information, the family/patient may be too shocked to give much verbal response. They may look dazed or withdrawn. With this reaction, hearing is limited and much repetition of information is needed. Similarly, anger can be a first reaction which usually dissipates with some passage of time. It is normal for patients and their families to be sad and express this feeling. Time and privacy should be provided to them.

Case Example 3

At 28 weeks Mr. and Mrs. W. had just learned that their singleton pregnancy was in fact twins and that each had a large encephalocele. When the social worker walked into the room to meet this couple, Mr. W. said: "Who are you and how can you possibly help us?" The social worker acknowledged their tremendous anxiety and sadness and anger. This defused the hostility so that the family was able to begin to look at the issues involved with their babies.

REINFORCEMENT OF DIAGNOSIS

Discussion of the actual diagnosis is best done in tandem with another health professional such as a perinatologist or geneticist. This can be done by having the social worker join the physician and family group during the actual testing procedure, and/or during the interview with the patient/family following the testing. Once the factual information has been given to the patient, further exploration of the issues surrounding the diagnosis can be explored by the social worker and the patient/family.

Comprehending medical explanations while coping with strong emotional feelings is very hard under the best of circumstances. When people are in shock or grieving, their coping mechanisms are often overwhelmed and information is not processed. Providing written information in a simple framework can help and should include the particular diagnosis and the available resource personnel. Such material augments the counseling process by allowing the patient and family to absorb information as they are able. Gathering the material ahead of time can facilitate the interviewing process.[2,3]

NONDIRECTIVE SUPPORT

The social worker and the family now begin to explore available options and resources. Linda Mealey,[4] writing in *Health and Social Work*, states that "the goal of a genetic counselor is to help clients reach a decision with which they can feel comfortable in the immediate and long-term future." She discusses constraints that all people face when making such hard decisions. During the interview, the social worker and family explore such constraints.

1. *Medical*–What are the known facts including the diagnosis and prognosis for this fetus and pregnancy?

Families will usually ask if there is any chance that the diagnosis could be wrong. An explanation of this particular problem and the testing procedure should again be given. The patient also often asks how the problem can be treated. More education and written materials can be used to demonstrate the available alternatives. For example, in the situation of a fetus with spina bifida, drawings may be used to indicate the level of the defect as well as using the ultrasound picture.

Case Example 4

A 17-year-old teen, accompanied by her grandfather, was seen at a local clinic for an ultrasound after an elevated AFP test. When the diagnosis of anencephaly was made, the patient was unable to comprehend the information and left the clinic. Her mother made another appointment at a large referral center where the social worker assessed the family's understanding of the anomaly while they waited for a second ultrasound. The patient asked questions such as whether her boy friend's drug use could have contributed to the problem and whether the anomaly could be fixed. By the time the patient had her ultrasound, they were more prepared for the diagnosis which they accepted as valid.

2. *Patient's motivation and personality*–What is the patient's age, level of intelligence, level of education and level of stress? Has the patient had a prior history with a similar problem? Has this resolved or is it ongoing? Is the patient fearful, shy, confident, hostile, etc.? How might the patient deal with the consequences of her decision? A young teen with little life experience may approach a problem differently than a mature woman with other children.

Case Example 5

A 36-year-old mother sought prenatal testing due to her age and her history of having a child with spina bifida from a previous relationship. The amniocentesis revealed a fetus with Down syndrome. The patient and her husband agonized over their decision, but finally elected to terminate the pregnancy. They felt that they could not handle an additional child with special needs, but were concerned that their daughter not feel rejected by their decision. The social worker encouraged this family to ventilate their feelings and gave suggestions for communicating their decision to their daughter. One year later this patient conceived and delivered a healthy baby.

3. *Patient's values*–Will the patient's religion affect this decision? How willing is the patient to take responsibility? What are her moral values?

Case Example 6

A young couple, who were students from an Asian country, faced a difficult decision when their fetus was found to have a chromosomal problem. They remarked that they would never be able to tell anyone from their family or culture about their decision to terminate a pregnancy, as it would be in conflict with their family's religious beliefs. They used the counseling session with the social worker to discuss their dilemma and guilt. Despite their cultural conflict, they were able to make a decision to terminate the pregnancy based upon their own circumstances and beliefs and in accord with each other.

4. *Family's values*–What family support is available to help? How strong is the relationship between the partners? Are there other children? How old are they? Has this couple experienced previous losses? If so, what were those losses?

Case Example 7

Mr. and Mrs. H. had a difficult pregnancy history. Their first pregnancy ended with a first trimester miscarriage. Mrs. H. next delivered a full-term stillborn daughter. Their next pregnancy was successful when their full-term son was born. In this, their fourth pregnancy, Mrs H.'s ultrasound revealed that the fetus had a diaphragmatic hernia. They were devastated, but decided to proceed with the pregnancy despite the poor prognosis as they felt they could deal with another loss. They maintained optimism throughout the pregnancy and used the counseling sessions to ventilate their ambivalence and anxiety. When their new daughter died several weeks after birth, this couple felt that the counseling and care they received had helped them get through another difficult experience with their marriage and family bruised but intact. Even in retrospect, they did not regret their decision to carry the pregnancy to term.

5. *Financial concerns*–How will this pregnancy and possible outcome affect the financial resources of this family? Will insurance or another third party payer be available? Who would be able to provide ongoing care for this child and would this necessitate a parent quitting a job? How will the cost of caring for the potentially handicapped child affect siblings and other family members?

The social worker can be instrumental in helping the family explore financial resources. Federal agencies such as the Bureau for Children with Medical Handicaps and the Rehabilitation Services Administration can help. State human service agencies and local agencies such as branches of the Easter Seal society can also provide assistance for eligible families. Other supportive resources are local groups focused on a particular diagnosis such as Down syndrome support groups or parents of children with spina bifida. Sometimes the social worker, with the permission of physician and patient, can introduce one family to another who has faced a similar problem.

Case Example 8 (See Case 3)

Mr. W., who was overwhelmed with sadness and anger at the dismal prognosis of his twin daughters, was also concerned about the financial burden and physical care that might need to be provided. With the social worker's guidance, he began to explore options for their care, should they survive. He visited local residential treatment facilities in his area and found out the cost of maintaining two babies at such an institution. Mr. W. discovered that the state could assume financial guardianship of the children, while he and his wife could pay a daily fee per child that was within their means. This research enabled him to begin to regain a sense of control and mastery.

6. *Legal and societal values*–Is this decision affected by the availability of termination or the availability of support services? At the current time, in most states, a pregnancy can only be terminated for non-lethal anomalies up to the 24th week of pregnancy. Often the time limit necessitates immediate decision-making under less than ideal conditions. The assessment process must be tailored to the individual needs of the patient and her level of comfort. As the variables are explored, often the patient and her family begin to express their concerns and their trend towards a particular decision or action, whether to continue or end the pregnancy.

INFORMATION AND ASSISTANCE
WITH TERMINATION PROCEDURE

Most families agonize over their decision-making and make their best decision based on the information and their particular circumstances. If the patient decides that abortion is her best option, counseling can help to reduce guilt. The social worker can emphasize two points that can help the patient. First, the worker can acknowledge the distinction between choosing to end a pregnancy for social reasons and making a decision to end a pregnancy because of knowledge of the poor fetal prognosis. Second, the worker can reduce the stigma of abortion by reassuring the patient that the health care team will support, be non-judgmental and remain available to the patient and her family.

The next step in the counseling process is an exploration and explanation of the availability of procedures. If comfortable and knowledgeable, the social worker can provide this information alone or with the physician or nurse. The social worker should be cognizant of resources for abortions at different gestational ages, i.e., abortion clinics, physicians available to provide abortions in their community and the financial requirements.

The types of termination procedures available for therapeutic reasons are based upon the gestational age of the fetus, the health of the mother, the availability of resources (agency, physician and/or hospital), the diagnosis and whether there is a need for postmortem or further genetic information and the patient's own preference.

Dilation and Suction Curettage (Suction D&C)

First trimester abortions are generally available as outpatient procedures in most communities. Until 12 weeks gestation, the fetus is small enough to be evacuated from the uterus with minimal dilation of the cervix, the narrow portion of the womb which opens into the vagina. This can be accomplished by mechanically dilating the cervix sufficiently to admit passage of a hard plastic tube called a suction curette (about 1 cm). The products of conception (fetus and placenta) are then extracted by an apparatus that vacuums them out of the uterus. This procedure can be performed in an outpatient setting under local anesthetic or in an ambulatory surgery setting if general anesthetic is requested. Tissue can be obtained for karyotyping or DNA or biochemical testing by experienced laboratories.

Dilation and Extraction (D&E)

Second trimester abortions are less widely available, are performed by fewer physicians and may require brief hospitalizations. After 12 weeks gestation the fetus is larger and evacuation of the uterus through the cervix is more difficult. Nonetheless, in the hands of an experienced physician, a D&E is the safest procedure for pregnancy termination up to 20 weeks gestation. To allow the cervix to dilate gradually and safely, several laminaria tents (slim pieces of special material which gradually expand as they absorb fluid) are placed into the cervix in the physician's office at least 6 hours before the D&E. The D&E is performed in an operating room, and patients usually receive a general anesthetic. Placenta and fetal parts are suctioned and mechanically extracted through the cervix. Tissue and even fetal blood can be obtained for further testing, but no recognizable fetus can be examined, making it more difficult to identify or confirm anomalies, nor can photographs be taken.

Many families prefer this type of termination procedure which ends the physical part of the pregnancy quickly. It is important to caution patients and their families that the grieving and mourning will not be as easily ended. They should be encouraged to gather mementoes of the pregnancy, such as ultrasound pictures, to remind them that the pregnancy and fetus did exist.

Induction of Labor

After 17 weeks, labor can be induced by placing prostaglandin suppositories into the vagina or by performing an amniocentesis to inject medicine, usually prostaglandin and/or urea into the uterus. This induces contractions and eventually a vaginal delivery of an intact fetus. As with a
D&E, laminaria tents must be placed into the cervix at the beginning of the
procedure to avoid tearing it at delivery. Though it sounds more invasive,
the injection procedure is usually best tolerated by the patient, as only one
injection is required, whereas the vaginal suppositories must be applied
repeatedly. The vaginal prostaglandin suppositories also have more side
effects: nausea, diarrhea and fever. During the induction, the patient experiences moderate cramping which becomes intense just before delivery.
Analgesics or epidural anesthesia can be given.

Though the procedure takes longer than a D&E, many families choose
the induction procedure because it leads to the birth of an intact fetus: a
tiny baby that they can acknowledge as a wanted child whom they have
lost because of its medical problems. In many cases it allows the family to
see the anomalies and validate their decision. It also allows a postmortem
examination to be performed which may be important in determining the
cause or recurrence risk of some fetal defects.

If at all possible, it is helpful for the social worker to visit the patient and
her family at the time of the abortion procedure. Referrals to other health
care professionals such as pastoral care, who also deal with grief and loss,
can be helpful. Once the abortion is completed, the patient and her family
should be cared for like any person who has miscarried a valued child.
With a D&E procedure, the patient will have few physical mementoes. If
available, an ultrasound picture should be offered. Other ways of memo-
rializing the pregnancy, like planting a tree or donating to a charity, can be
valuable to the patient. With an induction of labor and delivery, seeing,
holding, photographing and naming the baby should be offered and encouraged to promote the grieving and mourning process. Another aspect
of counseling is a follow-up sympathy card and phone call several days
after the termination. At this time, the social worker can ascertain whether
any unfinished business needs to be explored and the patient can further
ventilate her feelings.

Case Example 9

During the holiday season, a single young woman decided to terminate
her pregnancy, when at 22 weeks her fetus was found to have a bladder
obstruction with severe oligohydramnios. She underwent an induction of

labor on a floor that was normally not a gynecological area, where inexperienced nursing staff were working during the holidays. After this young woman delivered her baby, pictures were taken and put with the baby's footprints and other hospital mementoes. The day following the patient's discharge, the social worker called to offer support. She discovered that the patient was extremely upset as her packet with special memories of her baby and delivery was nowhere to be found. The worker went to the floor and questioned the nursing staff who had no idea where the packet might be as the chart had gone to medical records. The worker went to the patient's former room, found the packet in the bedside night table and called the patient with the news.

VALIDATION OF WORTH

Becoming pregnant and delivering a healthy baby are considered normal, natural and predictable events with a certain outcome. When a young woman and her partner are faced with a fetal problem and an uncertain outcome, it can be very damaging to their sense of self and trust. For the primiparous patient, such a diagnosis can be devastating. In addition to losing the hoped-for child, this patient and her partner are also facing the loss of their anticipated role as parents-to-be. Although the diagnosis cannot be changed, the patient and her partner will hopefully grow through the experience.

Case Example 10

Several years ago, a young couple came to a third medical center after being told at two other centers that their baby was anencephalic and that they should terminate the pregnancy at this gestational age of 20 weeks. Because they were not comfortable with this choice, they sought another option. The social worker counseled this family regarding choices at birth and ways to cope with the ongoing pregnancy and psychologically difficult birth experience. The young mother prepared for the birth of her baby by making a special hooded gown for the baby to wear and planning to have relatives present to see and be with the baby at delivery. The worker attended this delivery to provide support for this couple. When labor was induced at term, she survived several hours after delivery while surrounded by her caring parents and relatives. This couple was very appreciative of the care they received and returned to the same medical center and physician for care with two subsequent healthy pregnancies.

Working with families who must make a difficult decision for their unborn child challenges the skills and knowledge of the perinatal social worker. Helping these families survive this period can be extremely rewarding. The social worker in concert with the rest of the medical staff can help the patient regain a sense of control and mastery by treating her with respect and giving her as much information as possible. The goal for the counseling is to help this patient and her partner get through this difficult experience in the healthiest way. A team effort between the perinatal social worker and other health professionals can help promote this outcome.

Accepted for Publication: 05/15/96

NOTES

1. Van Putte, Alison. "Perinatal bereavement crisis: Coping with negative outcomes from prenatal diagnosis." *The Journal of Perinatal and Neonatal Nursing.* Vol II, No. 2. October, 1988.

2. Fertel, P., Iams, P. and Holowinsky, S. *Difficult Decisions.* Centering Corp., 1988.

3. Clark, S.L. and DeVors, G.R. "Clinical Commentaries: Prenatal diagnosis for couples who would not consider abortion." *Obstetrics and Gynecology. 73* (6): 1035-1037. 1988.

4. Mealey, L. "Decision making and adjustment in genetic counseling." *Health and Social Work. 9* (2). Spring, 1984.

BIBLIOGRAPHY

Adler, NE, David, HP, Major, BN et al.: Psychological responses after abortion. Science 248:41-44, 1990.

Berkowitz, RL, Lynch, L: Selective reduction: An unfortunate misnomer. Obstet Gynecol 75:873, 1990.

Blumberg, BD, Golbus, MS, Hanson, KH: The psychological sequelae of abortion performed for a genetic indication. Am J Obstet Gynecol 122:7 799-808, 1975.

Botkin, JR: Prenatal screening: The limits of parental choice. Obstet Gynecol 75:5 875-880, 1990.

Clark, SL, DeVors, GR: Clinical commentaries: Prenatal diagnosis for couples who would not consider abortion. Obstet Gynecol 73:6 1035-1037, 1988.

Colen, BD. *Hard Choices: Mixed Blessings of Modern Technology.* Putnam & Sons, NY, 1986.

Cullberg, J: Mental reactions of women to Perinatal death. Psych Med Obstet Gynaecol 3rd int. Congr., London 1971, 326-329, 1972.

Dagg, PKB: The psychological sequelae of therapeutic abortion performed for a genetic indication. Am J Psychiatry 148:5, 1991.

Elder, SH, Laurence, KM: The impact of supportive intervention after second trimester termination of pregnancy for fetal abnormality. Prenatal Diagnosis 2: 47-54, 1991.

Evans, MI, Drugan, A, Bottoms, SF et al.: Attitudes on the ethics of abortion, sex selection, and selective pregnancy termination among health care professionals, ethicists, and clergy likely to encounter such situations. Am J Obstet Gynecol 164:1092-1099, 1991.

Evans, MI, Fletcher, JC, Zador, IE et al.: Selective first-trimester termination in octuplet and quadruplet pregnancies: Clinical and ethical issues. Obstet Gynecol 71:3 289-296, 1988.

Fertel, PE, Iams, P, Holowinsky, S. *Difficult Decisions.* Centering Corp., Omaha, Neb., 1988.

Finley, SC, Varner, PD, Vinson, PC, Finley, WH: Participant's reaction to amniocentesis and prenatal genetic studies. JAMA 238:22 2377-2379, 1977.

Finnegan, J. *Shattered Dreams–Lonely Choices.* Bergin & Garvey, Westport, Conn., 1993.

Furlong, RM, Berkowitz, RL: Intrauterine treatment: Meeting the psychosocial needs of the family. Health Soc Work 10:55-63, 1985.

Greenfield, DA, Walther, VN: Psychological considerations in multifetal pregnancy reduction. Psychological Issues in Infertility 4:3 533-543, 1993.

Hobbins, JC: Selective reduction–a perinatal necessity? N Engl J Med 318: 1062-1063, 1988.

Ilse, S. *Precious Lives, Painful Choices: A Prenatal Decision-Making Guide.* Wintergreen Press, Maple Plain, Minn., 1993.

Kolata, G. *The Baby Doctors: Probing the Limits of Fetal Medicine.* Delacorte Press, New York, 1990.

Lynch, L, Berkowitz, RL, Chitkara, U et al.: First-trimester transabdominal multifetal pregnancy reduction: A report of 85 cases. Obstet Gynecol 76:215 735-738, 1990.

Mealey, L: Decision-making and adjustments in genetic counseling. Health Soc Work 9:2, 1984.

Notman, MT, Kravitz, AR, Payne, EC, Russell, JA: Psychological outcome in patients having therapeutic abortions. Psych Med Obstet Gynaecol 3rd int. Congr., London 1971, 552-554, 1972.

Rayburn, WF, LaFerla, JJ: Second-trimester pregnancy termination for genetic abnormalities. J Repro Med 27:9 584-588, 1982.

Rothman, BK. *The Tentative Pregnancy.* Penguin Books, New York, 1987.

Scully, T, Scully, C. *Making Medical Decisions.* Simon & Schuster, New York, 1989.

Van Putte, A: Perinatal bereavement crisis: Coping with negative outcomes from prenatal diagnosis. J Perinatal Neonatal Nursing 2:2, 1988.

Walther, VN: Emerging roles of social work in perinatal services. Soc Work in Health Care 15:2 35-48, 1991.

White-Van Mourik, MCA, Connor, JM, Ferguson-Smith, MA: Patient care before and after termination of pregnancy for neural tube defects. Prenatal Diag 10:497-505, 1990.

The Role of the Social Worker
in Perinatal Substance-Abuse

Cathy Cook, MSW

SUMMARY. Perinatal substance use affects approximately 10-15% of the population at any given time. Although it is not completely clear whether perinatal substance use is the cause of poor outcomes or a result of related factors such as poverty, environmental deprivation, violence in the home, or depression, the impact on maternal well-being and neonatal outcomes is enormous and the cost to society high. As this issue continues to receive state and national attention, the role for social workers as essential members of the treatment team is increasingly important. *[Article copies available for a fee from The Haworth Document Delivery Service: 1-800-342-9678. E-mail address: getinfo@haworth.com]*

INTRODUCTION

Maternal use of alcohol and other drugs is one of society's most significant contemporary problems. The National Institute of Drug Abuse (NIDA) Household Survey (1991) estimates that 27% of women between the ages of 18 and 25 have used illegal drugs within the past year and over six million have used alcohol. Moreover, NIDA (1991) estimates 9% of all women in childbearing years–ages 14 to 44–are current drug users. This may be an underestimate, because the NIDA National Household Survey does not provide good estimates of heavy drug use; it does not include

---

Cathy Cook is affiliated with Shands Hospital at the University of Florida.

[Haworth co-indexing entry note]: "The Role of the Social Worker in Perinatal Substance-Abuse." Cook, Cathy. Co-published simultaneously in *Social Work in Health Care* (The Haworth Press, Inc.) Vol. 24, No. 3/4, 1997, pp. 65-83; and: *Fundamentals of Perinatal Social Work: A Guide for Clinical Practice with Women, Infants, and Families* (ed: Regina Furlong Lind, and Debra Honig Bachman) The Haworth Press, Inc., 1997, pp. 65-83. Single or multiple copies of this article are available for a fee from The Haworth Document Delivery Service [1-800-342-9678, 9:00 a.m. - 5:00 p.m. (EST). E-mail address: getinfo@haworth.com].

persons who live in group quarters such as military installations, jails and prisons–persons likely to be heavy drug users. Estimates of use among pregnant women vary from 10 to 15% (100,000–375,000) of all pregnant women (Adams, Eyler, & Behnke, 1990).

The dramatic rise in drug-abusing parents has placed a serious strain both on the health care system and on an already overburdened child protective service system. The perinatal social worker often faces the dilemma of being between the chemically dependent prenatal or postnatal patient and the state child protective system. Judgment and skill are required to achieve balance between client advocacy and child protection where perinatal substance-abuse is a factor. Some of the most commonly abused drugs are: tobacco, alcohol, cocaine, marijuana, heroin and other opiates and prescription medications.

OBSTETRICAL COMPLICATIONS

The obstetrical complications associated with alcohol and other drug-abuse include spontaneous abortion, placental abruption, amnionitis, chorioamnionitis, breech presentation, gestational diabetes, intrauterine death, placental insufficiency, postpartum hemorrhage, eclampsia, preeclampsia, premature labor, premature rupture of membranes and septic thrombophlebitis (Miller & Hyatt, 1992).

The risk of HIV infection cannot be overstated. Drug use, with its ensuing sequelae such as poor nutrition, poor judgment, sleep deprivation and inadequate health care and housing, is believed to depress the immune system, making it more vulnerable to HIV and other infections (Department of Health and Human Services, 1990). Pregnancy itself is also associated with a suppression of immunity, especially during the last three months of pregnancy through up to three months after delivery. This decreased immunity increases a woman's susceptibility to infections, and it can make a pregnant woman more vulnerable to developing AIDS, especially if she is already seropositive (Centers for Disease Control, 1985). Common practices by vulnerable pregnant addicts, such as trading sex for drugs, unsafe sex, multiple partners, and needle-sharing can also increase the risk of contracting HIV and eventually AIDS. AIDS is one of the most devastating complications both for the woman and her fetus.

NEONATAL AND DEVELOPMENTAL COMPLICATIONS

It is difficult to analyze the effects of in utero exposure to specific substances, because the chemically dependent often abuse more than one substance. It is, however, now clear that the placenta is not a barrier for any substance (Lynch & McKeon, 1990). Infants suffering the most extreme effects are recognizable at birth, with approximately 18% requiring intensive care (Child Welfare League of America, 1992). In most cases, however, the effects of in utero exposure are much more subtle, and the newborn may present at birth with few or no symptoms at all. In fact, as many as 70% of these newborns may appear healthy; others may demonstrate mildly disorganized developmental patterns (Child Welfare League of America, 1992).

The range in severity of impairment is thought to be related to a number of prenatal factors including the type of drugs used, the characteristics of the drug (i.e., whether they were addictive, toxic, teratogenic, or a combination), the time and frequency of use, the general health and genetic history of the mother, and the amount of prenatal care (Child Welfare League of America, 1992). Paternal drug use may also be implicated (Gold, 1993). Among the drug use-associated complications of the neonate are respiratory distress syndrome, intrauterine growth retardation, autoimmune deficiency syndrome (AIDS), neonatal abstinence syndrome, hypocalcemia, intercranial hemorrhage, meconium aspiration, pneumonia, septicemia, hypoglycemia and hyperbilirubinemia (Miller & Hyatt, 1992). Children most at risk of impairment come from highly dysfunctional, heavily drug-involved families, where chemical abuse is only one of a multitude of problems.

The postnatal environment may, in fact, exacerbate or reduce existing problems. Environments where parents are chemically involved may pose a risk to the child in the form of abuse or neglect of health needs or nutrition (Child Welfare League of America, 1992). In addition, the infant's needs for attention, interaction and stimulation may not be met. In the worst case scenario, the infant is at risk for abuse, neglect, passive exposure to illicit drugs, and the chaos associated with drug use and community violence.

Even in the best environments, these infants may be difficult to care for and to nurture, particularly babies who are irritable, hypo- or hypersensitive to stimuli, sleep-disturbed, resistant to cuddling and prone to high-pitched screaming. Infants exposed prenatally to heroin or methadone may suffer ongoing vomiting and diarrhea. Children exposed to cocaine and other stimulants may exhibit feeding and sleep difficulties, excessive sucking, and poor weight gain (Howard's study [Cited in Child Welfare League of America, 1992]). Parents may have difficulty coping with and relating positively to infants who exhibit these behaviors. Researchers employing a range of diagnostic tools to assess drug-exposed infants have concluded that the behavior patterns of some affected neonates are likely to tax the ability of any caregiver to attach and respond positively to them (Howard & Beckworth, 1989). Thus, intervention strategies must counterbalance all of the interrelated factors that place the infant's development at risk.

As we observe the growth of children known to be prenatally exposed, concerns begin to emerge about the more subtle behaviors that may influence successful learning experiences and productive adult life. Some drug-exposed two-year-old children have been reported to have difficulty concentrating, interacting with others and coping with structured environments (Howard & Beckworth, 1989). It is not clear to what extent these characteristics are the result of prenatal exposure, low birthweight, inconsistent, inadequate care-giving, environmental deprivation, violence in the home, poverty, despair or other factors. The interplay between the prenatal and postnatal environments warrants further study.

SOCIAL WORK ASSESSMENT

The first and most important task for the perinatal social worker is the initial assessment. Prior to beginning this task, however, the perinatal social worker must conduct a personal values exploration and, in addition, learn about chemical dependency.

Some social workers enter the field of perinatal social work as a result of personal issues related to their own family of origin. These issues must be thoroughly examined for the potentiation of judgmental attitudes towards parents who abuse alcohol and other drugs. In the perinatal setting, it is especially important for the social worker to remain objective and nonjudgmental in assessing and intervening with substance-abusing families, since many other team members may feel justified regarding their own anger and punitive attitudes. Personal issues should not obfuscate the social worker's role as advocate and system liaison for the pregnant substance-abuser.

The social worker needs to understand the psychological, physical, social and family dynamics of addiction. Familiarity with the stages of addiction (including use, abuse and dependency, as well as resulting behavior and consequences) influences the services delivered and the type of intervention provided (e.g., legal, supportive, educational, etc.). A supportive educational approach could be used with individuals in the early use stage, whereas this approach would have little meaning for the client in the advanced stages of abuse.

Understanding the effects of various drugs and the significance of the terminology used in treatment of chemical dependency (i.e., dependency, tolerance, relapse, recovery, denial, enabling, codependency, etc.) will teach the social worker about the client's disease and also allow him/her to speak effectively with treatment providers and other professionals. Relationships with the treatment community that are based on trust and mutual respect will serve both the client and the social worker well.

An understanding of the process of relapse prevention and recovery process is critical, especially as it relates to the need for ongoing supports and aftercare services.

A written format is useful to provide the framework for the social work assessment of the chemically dependent patient. Such a format provides consistency to the interview and written documentation.

INTERVENTION

As with other health care problems, a comprehensive and coordinated approach to serving the needs of pregnant, chemically dependent women is necessary. Social workers, physicians, nurses and other health care providers must work as a team to identify the pregnant woman who has a substance-abuse problem. The perinatal social worker may serve as the team leader by initiating, coordinating and monitoring the multiple services needed by the chemically dependent pregnant woman. As case manager, the perinatal social worker not only engages the patient, but establishes the mechanisms to ensure cooperation and coordination from a variety of agencies, including child protection, financial assistance programs, educational systems, vocational programs and the legal and treatment communities.

The pregnant, chemically dependent woman brings multiple issues to social, health and welfare agencies, thus, coordinated gender-specific services are required. These multiple services include health and prenatal care, drug treatment, vocational training, child-care, parent education, assistance with survival needs such as food and housing, counseling for depression, low self-esteem, and isolation, and protection from abusive partners. These issues must always be addressed in any assessment and treatment plan.

TREATMENT ISSUES AND OPTIONS

Denial and self-deceit are key characteristics of addicts that must be confronted if any treatment is to be initiated. Cocaine abusers typically deny the severity of their addiction by romanticizing their relationship with the drug, thus minimizing its harmful effect on their lives (Washton, 1989). In the perinatal setting, the social worker may have the opportunity to confront the woman with her denial, pointing out any medical or behavioral indicators or contradictory statements. A positive toxicology screen either on the mother or the infant will lend much credence to this approach. Success in breaking through this denial is very often more indicative of the drug-abuser's stage of addiction and readiness to accept help than the clinical skills of the social worker (Millman, 1988).

A more time-intensive, family-systems, oriented approach would involve the family and determine the drug-abuser's role in the family system. Unfortunately, the use of denial in families of drug users is also common (Spitz & Spitz, 1987). From a family-systems perspective, the role of the drug-abuser may be to divert attention from other family problems (Stanton & Todd, 1982). Thus the social worker needs to evaluate the strengths and weaknesses of the drug-abuser's family, in order to determine which members of the family can best assist in confronting the addicts's use of denial (Spitz & Spitz, 1987).

The more people the social worker can involve in confronting the drug-abuser's denial, the greater the possibility that the person's defenses can be overcome, resulting in an immediate commitment to treatment (Spitz & Spitz, 1987). In an acute-care setting the health care team members, along with the family, can be a powerful force in helping the patient through the denial stage of her disease and into treatment (Gropper, 1991).

Once abuse is confirmed, the perinatal social worker faces some important decisions. Outpatient treatment is an inexpensive, less disruptive alternative for the motivated patient. But everyone is not a good candidate for outpatient treatment. Washton and Gold (1986) have suggested the following as criteria for inpatient treatment:

- Chronic freebase or intravenous use;
- Concurrent dependency on multiple drugs, including alcohol;
- Serious medical or psychiatric problems;
- Insufficient motivation for outpatient treatment;
- Lack of family and social supports;
- Failure in outpatient treatment.

Perinatal social workers are trained in a number of key areas that make them ideal practitioners in perinatal substance-abuse. The skills described by Carl Rogers over 30 years ago, including empathy for the concerns and aspirations of the client, acceptance of the client as a person worthy of regard, and a nonjudgmental attitude (Rogers, 1961), form the basis of a positive helping relationship with the pregnant substance-abuser. Miller et al. (1980) found that a therapist's empathy (as perceived by the client) is more predictive of problem drinkers' compliance with treatment goals than programmatic differences.

Another important influence on treatment outcome is confidence in one's skills. This self-confidence often emerges only after years of experience. But good supervision and continuing education can build skills and confidence quickly. A supportive peer network, such as a local group of perinatal social workers or substance-abuse treatment providers, can also enhance knowledge of resources and techniques, as well as mitigate against feelings of frustration and isolation.

Also crucial for success in working with substance-abusers is an ideology that permits flexibility of goal choice by the client or "self-determination," a familiar social work principle. The perinatal social worker's therapeutic skill is critical for appropriate goal setting and for recognizing the woman's strengths and weaknesses.

The availability of treatment will clearly influence outcome. A survey of treatment facilities in New York City (Harrison, 1991) showed that 87% had no beds for pregnant women on Medicaid. Of those treatment centers that did take pregnant women, only 44% made any type of child-care arrangements. Treatment does appear to improve neonatal outcomes; but its availability and adequacy are undocumented. Advocacy by the perinatal social worker for increases in available beds for pregnant and postpartum women is also an important function.

RACIAL/CULTURAL/GENDER ISSUES

Racial, cultural, and *gender issues* are critical in providing intervention and services to the chemically dependent pregnant or postpartum woman. Of the women arrested under expanded interpretation of child abuse and drug-trafficking statutes from 1988 to 1990, 80% were women of color (Paltrow et al., 1990). A recent Florida study by Chasnoff et al. (1990) conducted blind urine screens on nearly all women enrolled in prenatal care for a 6-month period, 380 women from the public health system and 335 women from the private sector. They found an overall incidence of 14.8% positive urine screens for alcohol, marijuana, cocaine and/or opiates. They found no significant differences in the rates from the public versus the private sector or white versus black populations. They did, however, find that the incidence of reporting substance-abusers to child protective services is 10 times greater for blacks than it is for whites (Chasnoff et al., 1990). Ninety-two percent of pregnant addicts who have been reported to authorities have incomes less than $25,000 (Chasnoff et al., 1990). Women are categorically discriminated against by treatment programs (Chavkin, 1990). Although 58% of drug addicts in the United States are women, women make up less than 30% of treatment admissions (Chavkin, 1990). The current system tends to blame the victim, often a poor woman of color, rather than providing appropriate, easily accessible treatment.

Although alcohol and other drug-abuse is not confined to one socioeconomic group, the specific needs of low-income women may be greater because of the lack of social and economic support available to them. These women are often isolated and involved in relationships with abusive men (Miller & Hyatt, 1992). There is a high correlation between substance-abuse and childhood physical and sexual abuse (Berenson et al., 1992; Swett et al., 1991). A poor, isolated parent with a history of abuse who may be using her infant to fulfill her own unmet needs is at high risk for child abuse. This risk will be increased by an irritable, unresponsive infant. In New York City, a study showed that 50% of child abuse and neglect cases brought before the court involved psychoactive substances and, if alcohol was included, the figure was 64% (Miller & Hyatt, 1992).

Since women are at the center of the issue of perinatal substance-abuse, *gender issues* must be addressed. A "double standard" exists for women in the area of substance-abuse, in that women are often stigmatized and considered "loose" or "easy" when using alcohol or other drugs. This stigma has a long history dating back to early Roman times, when Romulus forbade all drinking of alcohol by women–in the same measure that forbade adultery (Blume, 1990). Early historians (men) explained that women were forbidden to drink, because it caused them to be "sexually aggressive and promiscuous" (Blume, 1990). This ancient expectation has persisted in Western thought, as illustrated by some recent studies. George and colleagues (1986) had studied college students, shown videos and given written descriptions of dating scenarios. Women who ordered alcohol instead of soda were seen as more likely to engage in both foreplay and sexual intercourse. This perception was even more pronounced if a male paid for the drink.

In a similar study (George et al., 1986), women were asked if they became less particular regarding their choice of a sexual partner if they had been drinking. Defying the cultural stereotype, only 8% said yes, *and* 60% reported that a man who had been drinking had become sexually aggressive toward them. Richardson and Campbell (1982) showed college students videos of rape scenes that varied only as to who was intoxicated– the rapist or the victim. The viewers held the rapist less responsible if he had been drinking and the victim more responsible if she had been drinking. They viewed the woman as "less moral and more responsible" if she had been drinking. The stereotype that drinking and drugging equals promiscuity appears pervasive in society.

Why do women drink and take drugs? Much current evidence points to *depression* as the key; many women seem to be self-medicating a pervasive, underlying depression (Wilsnack, 1984; Wilsnack, 1989; Jacobson, 1989). In comorbidity studies involving diagnoses of alcoholism and depression, the primary diagnosis for men is alcoholism 78% of the time, but for women alcoholism is the primary diagnosis only 34% of the time (Helzer & Pryzbeck, 1988).

Much progress has been made in the area of women's treatment by Norma Finkelstein (1990) at the Coalition on Addiction, Pregnancy, and Parenting in Cambridge, Massachusetts. Building on the work of Carol Gilligan of Harvard and Jean Baker Miller and her colleagues at the Stone Center at Wellesley College (Gilligan, 1982; Miller, 1986), Finkelstein says that women are basically "relational beings," and that the traditional confrontational, isolating therapeutic techniques developed on middle-class men in the 1950s, may not work for women. The "Relational Model" recognizes that women develop a sense of self primarily through relationships or connections with others. Past, present and future connections are central to the development of self, which is a continuous process. Healthy relationships are defined as those that are mutually empowering–each person impacts the positive growth of the other. Finkelstein suggests building on women's unique strengths, such as the capacity for nurturing and the ability to connect with other human beings, by working with women in groups and encouraging them to support and nurture each other. Treatment must begin to help women take responsibility and avoid reinforcing passivity by reinforcing the assumption of traditional roles by males and females. Treatment that does not separate women from their children is also essential to maintain attachment and teach parenting skills.

LEGAL ISSUES

For the pregnant substance-abuser, the two legal issues with the most negative consequences are the *mandatory reporting* to child protection agencies of the delivery of a substance-exposed newborn and *prosecution* of the mother for child abuse or "delivering drugs" to a minor.

Mandatory reporting. The mandatory report is usually triggered by a positive toxicology screen for an illegal or prescription drug (excluding alcohol) at birth or, in some states, even admission of use during pregnancy. Child welfare advocates and state prosecutors have worked to have their child abuse statutes interpreted or amended to include prenatal substance-abuse, effectively declaring fetal rights.

Child welfare professionals tend to believe in mandatory testing and reporting of substance-abuse during pregnancy, because it puts them in contact with the families–ideally to provide essential support and services. Members of the legal community tend to want mandatory testing and reporting to both child protection agencies and state prosecutors, because they feel that the threat of prosection will keep women from using drugs. There is no clear data to prove that this is the case.

The goals of the more punitive approach are to protect both the unborn infant and the child following birth, assuming that a drug user cannot be an adequate parent and will abuse or neglect the child. The data on the relationship between child abuse and substance-abuse are somewhat suspect since they are derived primarily from correlations on families already heavily involved with the child welfare system (Murphy et al., 1991; Famularo et al., 1992). Although no one suggests that drug use or abuse contributes to positive parenting, it may not be appropriate to assume a mother will be a poor parent based on one factor. This approach is inconsistent with the way child welfare agencies have operated historically, using only acute events of abuse or neglect as reasonable cause to investigate. The Child Welfare League of America recommends that: "A parent's positive toxicology screen should not be the sole basis for a mandatory report to the child welfare authorities" (CWLA, 1992). A more appropriate use of a positive toxicology screen is as a risk factor to be included in a thorough psychosocial assessment used to determine the best way to support the mother and protect the child.

Toxicology screens. The majority of reports to both child protection agencies and prosecutors are based on a urine toxicology screen on either the mother or the infant. Toxicology screens raise a host of legal and ethical issues, the first of which is what exactly is measured. Toxicology screens do not measure frequency of drug use or impairment, nor do they necessarily predict neglectful parenting. Most drugs stay in the system for such a short period of time that only recent use is actually reflected in the screen. In addition, there is rarely a true "chain of custody," which is needed to protect evidence which may be used in court. Despite its unreliability, the toxicology screen leads to overreporting, thereby taxing the child welfare intake system. Further, it increases the risk of a newborn being removed from parents erroneously and placed in an overburdened foster care system. In turn this system may not adequately meet the child's needs (Coalition on Alcohol and Drug Dependent Women and Their Children, 1990).

Who should receive toxicology screens and who makes this decision? It is unclear whether all pregnant women and newborns should be the subject of screening or only those whom the physician suspects may have used or been exposed to illicit drugs. Universal screening is expensive and is a questionable use of limited resources. Selective screening, however, seems to be discriminatory, since medical providers at public facilities may be more likely to use screens than their counterparts at private hospitals (Gustavsson, 1992). And even within the public facilities, poor minority women are tested at a higher rate (Graven, 1989).

In addition, many physicians feel conflicted about their role as health care providers when they order specific tests for legal rather than medical reasons. The health care provider has not traditionally been viewed as an agent of the government. This can also be difficult for the perinatal social worker who may be encouraged by the child protection agency to press for a screen to be ordered. This may conflict with her/his role as a member of the health care team and as a helping professional (Moseley & Bell, 1991). The perinatal social worker must always consider the importance of a positive toxicology screen on a perinatal patient. She must consequently initiate the full assessment of the parents' alcohol and other drug use and its impact on their ability to protect and nurture the child. And if the assessment establishes a basis for the suspicion of abuse of neglect, the worker must file a report with child protective services. It is important to inform the mother that such a report is being made and what the process and ramifications are.

Informed consent and confidentiality of medical information are critical issues. Women rarely give informed consent for testing for themselves or their infants. The information obtained from the screen is then transferred without their knowledge or consent to state attorneys pursuing prosecution. Over the past several years, state prosecutors have used this information to apply a variety of laws, such as child abuse, criminal possession, and delivery of illegal substances, and assault to punish women who engage in alcohol and other drug-abuse while pregnant (Coalition on Alcohol and Drug Dependent Women and Their Children, 1990).

Prosecution. It is estimated 164 women in 24 states have been arrested over the last five years on criminal charges resulting from their drug-related behavior while pregnant or because they became pregnant while addicted to drugs (Paltrow, 1992). The majority of these cases have been concentrated in South Carolina or Florida. In July 1989, a trial court in Florida convicted Jennifer Johnson of "delivering drugs" to her newborn via the placenta in the 60 to 90 seconds after birth but before the umbilical cord was severed (Coalition on Alcohol and Drug Dependent Women and

Their Children, 1990). In July of 1992, the case was overturned by the Florida Supreme court (Paltrow, 1992). This, along with another over-turned conviction in South Carolina, may reflect legal and public policy arguments that prosecution is counterproductive and dangerous, driving women away from prenatal care.

In 1990, the Coalition on Alcohol and Drug Dependent Women and Their Children drafted resolutions opposing both mandatory reporting and prosecution. The resolution against mandatory reporting was signed by 14 national organizations, including the American Civil Liberties Union, the American College of Nurse-Midwives, The National Perinatal Association and the National Association of Perinatal Social Workers. The resolution opposes "non-consensual testing and reporting of medical records revealing drug use by pregnant women to prosecutors as evidence of child abuse or neglect or criminal behavior" (1990). The resolution on prosecution states,

> We . . . oppose criminal prosecution of alcohol- and drug-dependent women solely because they were pregnant when they used alcohol or drugs. The threat of criminal prosecution prevents many women from seeking prenatal care and early intervention for their alcohol or drug dependence, undermines the relationship between health and social service workers and their clients, and dissuades women from providing accurate and essential information to health care provid-ers. The consequence is increased risk to the health and development of their children and themselves. (1990)

Perinatal social workers must advocate both for women and their in-fants in the child welfare and legal system. As part of the assessment, social workers help determine safety for the infant at discharge. Based on this crucial role, some hospitals use the social worker as the team leader in a multi-disciplinary approach to the problem. The social worker is usually familiar with reporting policies and procedures to local child protection authorities and often has a relationship with the agency. Thorough social work documentation lends credibility to the assessment, reporting and treatment referral process. It is through comprehensive treatment includ-ing prenatal and child care, not criminalization, that women can overcome their alcohol and drug dependence and safely rear their children.

Staff Attitudes

The inherent dilemma for the perinatal social worker as well as other health care staff is that there are two patients, one of whom cannot speak for itself. This becomes especially poignant for all staff when the patient refuses treatment for addiction, yet has an infant to care for or is perhaps still pregnant and using drugs. The image of damaged fetuses arouses our compassion and concern. Our frustration in solving the problem of drug addiction in pregnancy and protecting the fetus from harm, drives us to solutions that identify the woman as the cause. In our haste, we may find ourselves responding to our need to "do something." We may rely on questionable data. We may turn to solutions that defeat the ultimate and legitimate purpose of caring for the woman and protecting the fetus. An adversarial relationship between the mother and the fetus works to no one's advantage. In order to begin to resolve the dilemma, it is useful to look at several aspects of the problem, including emotional reactions of helpers, the validity of information used in decision-making and the issue of identification (Harrison, 1991).

Personal *emotional* reactions are difficult to assess. In order to work successfully with addicted pregnant patients, we must be honest with ourselves, both as social workers and as human beings. Do these cases anger, sadden, disgust us? What is our ideology? Do we believe that the fetus is a person with the same rights as the mother? Twenty years ago this conflict between the mother and the fetus was unheard of. There was a general assumption that the pregnant woman had the best interest of her baby at heart. There now appears to be a trend toward mistrust of the pregnant woman's ability to care for her unborn infant. As perinatal social workers, we need to honestly identify our feelings and attitudes about pregnancy and the responsibility it entails, and then sensitize ourselves to the needs of both the mother and her infant.

Information on perinatal substance-abuse also influences attitudes. Much of the data on pregnant substance-abusers are inconsistent and vary greatly depending on the method and the demographic characteristics of the population. These data are quoted as factual and used as justification for both institutional and broader social policy. These policies in turn determine which social, political and legal interventions with mothers and babies are acceptable.

Many of the perinatal outcome data related to poverty are the same as for perinatal substance use—intrauterine growth retardation (IUGR), low birth weight (LBW), etc. Perhaps polydrug use could be seen as one symptom of poverty, along with poor nutrition, violence, lack of support, despair and stress. These data then might be used to support social policy and subsidize intervention to improve the life of the woman rather than restrict it.

In a study by Koren et al. (1989), it was found that the research (primarily unpublished) which showed negative results was just as valid as that showing positive results. This bias against negative results also discourages researchers from doing the kind of research that might not show differences between groups. Thus, research which showed little difference between substance-exposed and non substance-exposed infants would be less likely to be published. Publishing, in its control of reported data, also controls what is defined as truth (Harrison, 1991). In addition, there are few studies of middle- and upper-middle-class addicted women. While routine screening may occur with indigent populations, it is rare among private middle-class patients. Information gathering is a step in creating social policy that must be reevaluated constantly in terms of its reliability, meaning and applicability. These issues should frame the questions that perinatal social workers and other health care professionals ask when making decisions about mothers, babies or agency policy.

Social workers need to examine *identification* (Harrison, 1991). We now know that the placenta does not serve as a barrier (Lynch & McKeon, 1990). Technology has made the fetus much more readily available through ultrasound and fetal monitoring, for example. Also, the abortion debate has also contributed to the "shift of allegiance" in obstetrics. The shift is evident even in the change in terminology from obstetrics to perinatology to maternal/fetal medicine. The perinatal social worker must be vigilant in maintaining a social work identity rather than aligning with the perinatal or neonatal medical service. The fetus remains vulnerable and unseen and lacks the social class and ethnic distinction which make identification with the mother so difficult. In large public and teaching hospitals, the backgrounds of the patients and the staff are often radically different. Further, substance-abusing patients are doing something illegal and self-destructive. Many may not have sought prenatal care and are seen as lacking in concern for the fetus. Generally, they are not easy to care for and we hold them responsible for their actions. Even professionals often see their actions from the standpoint of the taxpayer–"supporting those women." It is important to be conscious of this process of identification, both in ourselves and in other caretakers, as we struggle to provide care and make crucial decisions.

Ethics

Two key principles inform our ethical views on perinatal substance-abuse: beneficence and autonomy. Beneficence is defined in the Hippocratic oath, "do no harm." In its more current form, Beauchamp and Childress (1994) argue that beneficence "asserts an obligation to help others further their important and legitimate interests." Providing benefit to the patient, as defined by their own values, is generally assumed to be the goal of health care (Beauchamp & Childress, 1994). Even this straightforward principle becomes complex in the case of the perinatal substance-abuser, because there are two separate patients in one body, with possibly different and conflicting interests. The ethical question becomes, whose interests or welfare should prevail? This dilemma is not resolved simply by following well-meaning yet ill-conceived state screening requirements and politically motivated charges of child abuse. An acceptable resolution that protects the interests of both the pregnant woman and the fetus might support the use of prenatal drug screening for diagnostic and therapeutic purposes only. Yet the perinatal social worker must in reality, determine which patient receives the highest priority in terms of therapeutic intervention. This is especially difficult for the perinatal social worker who is charged with making the best discharge plan for the newborn infant. To whom does he/she owe allegiance? Based on the historic role of social workers in child protection, her/his first allegiance must be to the infant, who cannot protect herself from harm. The second priority is to find appropriate treatment and services for the mother, who is motivated to enhance her ability to provide good nurturing care for her infant.

In grappling with such a difficult issue, it can be helpful to look to the ethical principle of autonomy which is necessary to provide a limit on beneficence (Gauthier, 1990). Beauchamp and Childress (1994) discuss autonomy in terms of actions that are intentional, understood and carried out while "remaining free from controlling interferences by others." Accordingly, in a health care setting, fully competent patients and clients should be making the decisions concerning their own treatment, free from interference from the health care staff (Gauthier, 1990). Thus, during pregnancy, the woman is the primary decision-maker. As previously mentioned, self-determination (patient autonomy) is an important and ingrained social work value, with exercise of choice as an important component.

This issue of women's freedom of choice is raised for the perinatal social worker when pregnant women are prosecuted and jailed for simple use of illegal drugs, when other nonpregnant people are not. Is it ethical to restrict lifestyle choices of pregnant women more than those who are not pregnant? Consider whether this limitation of the freedom of pregnant women could be applied to other lifestyle choices as well, such as the use of legal drugs known to be harmful to the fetus (i.e., alcohol, tobacco, caffeine, aspirin). What about flying in an airplane or engaging in certain types of exercise? Drawing a line regarding self-governance is an awesome responsibility. The perinatal social worker must use extreme caution in being a part of any act that supports autonomy for fetuses at the expense of the mother.

Children who are already born, however, are another matter, and if the mother's pursuit of her own autonomy endangers her child, it should be reported according to specific state statutes. One ethicist has said, "At the very root of ethics, there is a tension. It springs from the difference between respecting the freedom and securing the best interests of persons" (Englehardt, 1986). This is especially poignant when there are two persons' autonomy and best interests to consider.

In a health care setting operating under the medical model, it may be acceptable for health care providers to arbitrarily decide what are the best interests of the patient, while ignoring the patient's right to self-determination. The perinatal social worker is in the best position to advocate for the autonomy of the patient and mitigate against an all-too-prevalent paternalistic attitude on the part of health care staff. This is a situation in which the principle of autonomy can be used to limit beneficence which has become paternalistic.

In addition to advocating for the individual woman and her infant, the perinatal social worker works for more ethical policy on an institutional, community, state and national level. The social worker has the knowledge and the expertise about perinatal substance-abuse to make a credible argument for needed policy changes.

CONCLUSION

Substance use among pregnant women has received increased public attention in recent years. That in itself is an interesting phenomenon, in view of the fact that it is not a new problem. For as long as humans have been using and abusing alcohol and other drugs, women have been conceiving and delivering babies. Maternal chemical use represents one important risk factor among many others. A multiple-risk model can provide guidance for needs assessment and intervention. The likelihood of negative perinatal outcome may be proportional to the number of risk factors. The perinatal social worker is in the ideal position to assess the whole person in her environment and present recommendations to the multidisciplinary team. This is both an opportunity and an important responsibility for the perinatal social worker.

Accepted for Publication: 05/15/96

REFERENCES

Adams, C., Eyler, F. & Behnke, M. (1990). Nursing intervention with mothers who are substance abusers. *Journal of Perinatal and Neonatal Nursing, 3*(4), 43-52.

Beauchamp, T. & Childress, J. (1994). *Principles of biomedical ethics.* New York: Oxford University Press.

Berenson, A., Sand Miguel, V. & Wilkinson, G. (1992). Violence and its relationship to substance use in adolescent pregnancy. *Journal of Adolescent Health, 13*, 470-474.

Blume, S. (1990). Alcohol and drug problems in women. In H. Milkman & L. Sederer (Eds.), *Treatment choices for alcoholism and substance abuse* (pp. 183-200). Lexington, MA: Lexington Books.

Centers for Disease Control. (1985). Recommendations for assisting in the prevention of perinatal transmission of HTLV/HIV and AIDS. *Morbidity and Mortality Weekly Report, 34*, 721-732.

Chasnoff, I., Landress, H. & Barrett, M. (1990). Prevalence of illicit drug and alcohol use in Pinellas county, Florida, and discrepancies in mandatory reporting. *New England Journal of Medicine, 322*, 1202-1206.

Chavkin, W. (1990). Drug addiction and pregnancy: Policy crossroads. *American Journal of Public Health, 80*(4), 483-487.

Child Welfare League of America. (1992). *Children at the front: A different view of the war on alcohol and drugs.* Washington, DC: Child Welfare League of America, Inc.

Coalition on Alcohol and Drug Dependent Women and Their Children. (1990). *Resolution on mandatory reporting.* Washington, DC: National Council on Alcoholism and Drug Dependence.

Coalition on Alcohol and Drug Dependent Women and Their Children. (1990). *Resolution on prosecution.* Washington, DC: National Council on Alcoholism and Drug Dependence.

Coalition on Alcohol and Drug Dependent Women and Their Children. (1990). *State legislative and policy proposals.* Washington, DC: Author.

Englehardt, H. (1986). *The foundations of bioethics.* New York: Oxford University Press.

Famularo, R., Kinscherff, R. & Fenton, T. (1992). Parental substance abuse and the nature of child maltreatment. *Child Abuse and Neglect, 16*, 475-483.

Finkelstein, N. (1990). *Treatment issues: Women and abuse.* Prepared for the Coalition on Alcohol and Drug Dependent Women and Their Children, Washington, DC.

Gauthier, C. (1990). Ethical issues in perinatal social work. *NAPSW Forum, 10*(4), 6-9.

George, W., Skinner, J. & Marlatt, G. (1986). Male perceptions of the drinking woman: Is liquor quicker? Paper presented at the meeting of the Eastern Psychological Association, New York, April.

Gilligan, C. (1982). *In a different voice.* Cambridge, MA: Harvard University Press.

Gold, M. (1993). *Cocaine.* New York: Plenum Medical Book Company.

Graven, M. (1989). *Maternal drug-use project summary.* Unpublished research, University of Florida.

Gropper, M. (1991). The many faces of cocaine: The importance of psychosocial assessment in diagnosing and treating cocaine abuse. *Social Work in Health Care, 16*, 97-111.

Gustavsson, N. (1992). Drug exposed infants and their mothers: Facts, myths, and needs. *Social Work in Health Care, 16*, 87-100.

Harrison, M. (1991). Drug addiction in pregnancy: The interface of science, emotion and social policy. *Journal of Substance Abuse Treatment, 8*, 261-268.

Helzer, J. & Pryzbeck, T. (1988). The co-occurrence of alcoholism with other psychiatric disorders in the general population and its impact on treatment. *Journal of Studies on Alcohol, 49*, 219-224.

Howard, J. & Beckworth, L. (1989). The development of young children of substance abusing parents: Insights from seven years of intervention and research. *Zero to Three, 9*(5), 8-12.

Jacobson, G. (1989). Alcohol and drug dependency problems in special populations: Women. In G. Larson & A. Larson (Eds.), *Alcoholism and substance abuse in special populations* (pp. 385-404). Rockville, MD: Aspen Publishers.

Koren, G., Graham, K., Shear, H. & Einarson, T. (1989). Bias against the null hypothesis: The reproductive hazards of cocaine. *Lancet, 2*, 1440-1442.

Lynch, M. & McKeon, V. (1990). Cocaine use during pregnancy. *Journal of Obstetric, Gynecological, and Neonatal Nursing, 19*, 285-292.

Miller, J. (1986). *Toward a new psychology of women.* Boston: Beacon Press.

Miller, W. & Hyatt, M. (1992). Perinatal substance abuse. *American Journal of Drug and Alcohol Abuse, 18*, 247-261.

Miller, W., Taylor, C. & West, J. (1980). Focused versus broad-spectrum behavior therapy for problem drinkers. *Journal of Clinical and Consulting Psychology, 48*, 590-601.

Millman, R. (1988). Evaluation and clinical management of cocaine abusers. *Journal of Clinical Psychiatry, 49* (suppl), 27-33.

Moseley, R. & Bell, C. (1991). Prenatal screening for illegal drugs. *Journal of Nurse-Midwifery, 36*, 245-248.

Murphy, J., Jellinek, M., Quinn, D., Smith, G., Poitrast, G. & Goshko, M. (1991). Substance abuse and serious child mistreatment: Prevalence, risk, and outcome in a court sample. *Child Abuse and Neglect, 15*(3), 197-211.

National Institute on Drug Abuse. (1991). *National household survey on drug abuse: Population estimates 1991.* Rockville, Maryland, U.S. Department of Health and Human Services.

Paltrow, L. (1992). *Criminal prosecutions against pregnant women,* Monograph, American Civil Liberties Union Reproductive Freedom Project, New York.

Paltrow, L., Fox, H. & Goet, E. (1990). *Memorandum,* American Civil Liberties Union Reproductive Freedom Project, New York.

Richardson, D. & Campbell, J. (1982). Alcohol and rape: The effects of alcohol on attributions of blame for rape. *Personality and Social Psychology Bulletin, 8*, 468-476.

Rogers, C. (1961). Formulation of the person and the social contract. In S. Koch (Ed.), *Psychology: A study of a science, Vol. III.* (pp. 184-256). New York: McGraw-Hill.

Spitz, H. & Spitz, S. (1987). Family therapy of cocaine abusers. In H. Spitz &

J. Rosecan (Eds.), *Cocaine abuse: New directions in treatment and research* (pp. 202-232). New York: Brunner/Mazel.

Stanton, M., & Todd, T. (1982). *The family therapy of drug abuse and addiction.* New York: Guilford Press.

Swett, C., Cohen, C., Surrey, J., Compaine, A. & Chavez, R. (1991). High rates of alcohol use and history of physical and sexual abuse among women outpatients. *American Journal of Drug and Alcohol Abuse, 17*(1), 49-60.

United States Department of Health & Human Services. (1990). Alcohol & Health. Rockville, MD.

Washton, A. (1989). *Cocaine addiction: Treatment, recovery, and relapse prevention.* New York: W.W. Norton and Company.

Washton, A. & Gold, M. (1986). *Cocaine treatment: A guide.* Rockville, MD: American Council for Drug Education.

Wilsnack, S. (1984). Drinking, sexuality, and sexual dysfunction in women. In C. Wilsnack & L. Beckman (Eds.), *Alcohol problems in women: Antecedents, consequences, and intervention* (pp. 189-227). New York: Guilford.

Wilsnack, S. (1989). Drinking, and drinking problems in women: A U.S. longitudinal survey and some implications for prevention. In T. Loberg, W. Miller, P. Nathan & G. Marlatt (Eds.), *Addictive behaviors: Prevention and early intervention* (pp. 117-138). Amsterdam: Swets & Zeitlinger.

Perinatal Social Work
with Childbearing Adolescents

Diane Adams, MSW
Susan M. Kocik, MSW

SUMMARY. Issues relating to adolescent childbearing have rapidly moved to the forefront of this nation's agenda. The implications of an adolescent's decision to have a baby have health, social and economic consequences for the adolescent, her offspring, partner and family and for all of society. This article will discuss the health, social and developmental consequences of adolescent childbearing and provide an overview of social work practice with childbearing adolescents. *[Article copies available for a fee from The Haworth Document Delivery Service: 1-800-342-9678. E-mail address: getinfo@haworth.com]*

One million adolescents in the United States are expected to become pregnant by the end of this year (Alan Guttmacher Institute: 1988). If the recent past is any indication of the present, by the end of this day approximately 3,013 teenagers will have conceived (Rich: 1991). About half of these teenagers will, for a variety of reasons, choose to carry their pregnancies to term and face the irrevocable, monumental, lifetime task of parenthood. The health, social and economic consequences of this decision impacts not only the teen parent but also her offspring, partner, family

Diane Adams is Adolescent Pregnancy Social Worker at The Mount Sinai Medical Center, 1 Gustave Levy Place, P.O. Box 1252, New York, NY 10029. Susan M. Kocik is Social Service Coordinator at The Hemophelia Program, Puget Sound Blood Center, 921 Terry Avenue, Seattle, WA 98104.

[Haworth co-indexing entry note]: "Perinatal Social Work with Childbearing Adolescents." Adams, Diane, and Susan M. Kocik. Co-published simultaneously in *Social Work in Health Care* (The Haworth Press, Inc.) Vol. 24, No. 3/4, 1997, pp. 85-97; and: *Fundamentals of Perinatal Social Work: A Guide for Clinical Practice with Women, Infants, and Families* (ed: Regina Furlong Lind, and Debra Honig Bachman) The Haworth Press, Inc., 1997, pp. 85-97. Single or multiple copies of this article are available for a fee from The Haworth Document Delivery Service [1-800-342-9678, 9:00 a.m. - 5:00 p.m. (EST). E-mail address: getinfo@haworth.com].

and society as a whole. The following is meant as a general overview of perinatal social work with childbearing adolescents.

EPIDEMIOLOGY

Given the well documented adverse effects of adolescent childbearing and the increasingly high cost of programs serving these adolescents, there is heightened public interest in the number of teen pregnancies and births. Some may find solace in the declining birth rate among adolescents from the mid 1970s to 1990. However, when the following factors are taken into account, this decline becomes less significant: (1) the United States has the highest adolescent birth rates when compared to other developed countries (specifically Canada, England and Wales, France, the Netherlands and Sweden) (Child Welfare League of America: 1995), (2) because there has been a more drastic decline in the birthrate in the non-adolescent population, the proportion of adolescent births to total births has increased, (3) although the birth rate has decreased, the number of aborted pregnancies by adolescents has increased, (4) the actual adolescent population has decreased (Zabin & Hayward: 1993), (5) the birth rate among young adolescents has not mirrored that of the older adolescents and has steadily increased (Encyclopedia of Social Work: 1987) and (6) most recent data shows that the birth rate for middle adolescents (15-17 years old) has increased from 1986 to 1988 by 10% (Alan Guttmacher Institute: 1988), and from 1980-1992 by 18.2%.

As concern about adolescent childbearing increases, and as prevention of adolescent pregnancy slowly moves to the forefront of this nation's agenda, many professionals have postulated possible explanations for the high pregnancy and birth rate. Focus has been on the ineffective, inconsistent or lack of contraceptive use among many adolescents and the myriad of variables that contribute to this. Barriers to effective contraceptive use include: lack of knowledge or misconceptions about reproduction and contraception; fear or embarrassment that their sexual activity will be discovered; unexpected and unplanned intercourse; and difficulty negotiating various systems needed to obtain birth control. Another variable in the contraceptive equation (especially among younger adolescents) is the adolescent's cognitive level. Adolescents are just beginning the transition from concrete operational thought to formal operational thought and may be less able to think abstractly (Piaget: 1972, Jorgenson: 1983). In addition, much of the adolescent's behavior may be driven by what Elkind (1988) describes as the "personal fable," an adolescent's belief in his or her invulnerability.

Although adolescent childbearing spans all races and socioeconomic groups, an adolescent mother is most likely to be from a background of poverty and disadvantage (Hayes: 1987, Leland: 1987, Scholl et al.: 1984). Upon noting this large percentage of poor, inner-city minority teens electing to raise their children, some have questioned whether the decision to become a mother is a response to a sense of alienation, isolation and a lack of future opportunities. Therefore, although research indicates that 70-90 percent of pregnancies are unplanned, there are a growing number of clinicians who believe that, at some level, more of these pregnancies were planned, or at least deliberately not prevented. "In a nation where one's worth is judged primarily in three areas–school, work, and family–it is not surprising that teenagers who cannot find a way to succeed in the first two areas find no reason to delay resorting to the third" (The Children's Defense Fund: 1986).

In a study focusing on teenagers who are willing to consider out of wedlock childbearing, Abrahamse, Morrison and Waite concluded that teenagers with more self-reported school discipline and truancy problems were more likely to consider childbearing (1988). Teenagers with higher educational expectations, and thus perhaps a more positive outlook on their opportunities, were least likely to consider childbearing. Dash (1989) sadly concluded that it is the "poor academic preparation . . . , the poverty that surrounds them, the social isolation from mainstream American life that motivates many of these boys and girls to have children." It is apparent that there is no simple explanation that can be isolated to be responsible for the high adolescent birth rate in the United States.

BIOPSYCHOSOCIAL IMPLICATIONS

The phrase "adolescence" is from the Latin word "adolescere" which means to grow up. G. Stanley Hall described this growing up period between childhood and adulthood as a time of "storm and stress." While in recent years practitioners have challenged whether adolescence needs to be characterized by such storm and stress, clearly it is a time of rapid change in almost all areas of life.

Much attention and research in the United States and in other developed countries have focused on the consequences of superimposing pregnancy, a normative crisis in a woman's lifetime, on adolescence, a period of rapid, all encompassing growth. It has been generally accepted, and only recently challenged, that teenage childbearing increases the biological, sociological and psychological risks to both mother and baby and leads to a lifetime of poverty and welfare dependence.

HEALTH CONSEQUENCES OF EARLY CHILDBEARING

The health consequences and pregnancy outcomes of early childbearing have been studied and cited frequently. It has been found that adolescents are at higher risk for: anemia; pre-eclampsia; poor pregnancy weight gain; low birth weight; cervical trauma; premature delivery; and infant death (Nichols: 1991, Center for Population Options: 1991). Some studies have questioned whether it is maternal age that places these adolescents at risk or other variables that are associated with adolescent childbearing such as the effects of poverty (Makinson: 1985), little or no prenatal care (Young et al.: 1989) and/or poor nutritional habits (Scholl et al.: 1984). Recent studies which controlled for socioeconomic variables concluded that there may be a biological basis for the increased health risks among pregnant adolescents (Fraser, Brockert, & Ward: 1995).

SOCIAL IMPLICATIONS

Lockhart and Wodarski (1990) write: "Adolescents who become pregnant are ensuring for themselves and their babies a future marked by truncated education, inadequate vocational training, poor work skills, economic dependency and poverty, large single parent households, and social isolation." As mentioned previously, since this nation is experiencing difficult economic times, society at large has expressed grave concerns over the cost of early childbearing, especially through programs such as AFDC and WIC (Burt: 1986). The notion that the social implications for young women who choose childbearing must always be bleak is beginning to be challenged (Buchholz & Gol: 1986, Furstenberg, Brooks-Gunn, & Morgan: 1987). While acknowledging that early childbearing places the adolescent and her child at a disadvantage in most areas of her life, there are an increasing number of studies indicating that some teenagers are overcoming these disadvantages. Just as there is considerable diversity in the population of childbearing adolescents, so there is significant variability in their lives as mothers. Researchers, in examining the variability of early childbearing outcomes, are attempting to discern the variables that increase the likelihood a young mother will overcome disadvantage. Furstenberg, in his landmark study of adolescent mothers in later life, examined the variables that increased the likelihood that, seventeen years after the birth of her first child, a mother would be receiving welfare and would have three or more children. The adolescent's level of education, both prior to and after her first child, had a direct impact on the likelihood of her overcoming some of the disadvantages of early childbearing (Furstenberg, Brooks-Gunn, & Morgan: 1987).

When addressing the social implications of adolescent childbearing, it is difficult to isolate pregnancy from other aspects of the adolescent's life. For some of these teens, the pregnancy is just a symptom of an already disadvantaged chaotic life. Continuing to examine the factors that increase the likelihood of positive well-being for both young mothers and their children will allow social workers to target those adolescents who are in need of more intense social work involvement and, it is hoped, will lead to more effective interventions.

PSYCHOLOGICAL/DEVELOPMENTAL IMPLICATIONS

Recently, attention has been given to the dual developmentalism of the childbearing adolescent (Barr & Monserrat: 1992; Hamburg: 1986; Sadler & Catrone: 1983). The pregnant and parenting teen is first and foremost an adolescent who is working, perhaps struggling, through the tasks of early, middle and late adolescence and gradually assuming more autonomous, adult roles. The adolescent moves from concrete operational thought to formal operational thought; begins to develop her own identity; experiments with what she perceives to be adult behaviors; and strives for autonomy and independence from her family. She may have a heightened need for peer acceptance and may be both narcissistic and egocentric (Sadler & Catrone: 1983, Barr & Monserrat: 1992). While much is contingent upon the adolescent's age, past experience and maturity, the tasks of pregnancy and parenting may be diametrically opposed to the tasks of adolescent development. Therefore it is crucial for perinatal social workers to assess the adolescent's stage of development (i.e., what tasks has she mastered and what characteristics are prominent?) and identify potential areas of conflict (i.e., will the adolescent be able to place the needs of her baby over her own? Will she be able to plan for the future?).

IMPLICATIONS FOR SOCIAL WORK PRACTICE

The extent of, and indications for, social work involvement will vary depending upon the adolescent's and the social worker's assessment of needs. Social work involvement may include help with public assistance, help with school or with day care, support of the teen in notifying her family and/or significant other of the pregnancy and exploration of ambivalence with the decision to raise the baby and review of available options (such as abortion and adoption). Child protective issues as well as issues relating to homelessness, HIV infection, sexual abuse, physical abuse, depression and past losses may arise. While the sheer volume of most social workers' case loads necessitates prioritizing, neither the provision of concrete services nor more traditional psychotherapy or counseling should be devalued.

Each childbearing teen brings to the pregnancy unique past experiences which will directly affect both her ability to cope with the pregnancy and her potential for positive parenting. A thorough comprehensive assessment of the adolescent's strengths, needs and developmental stage is essential. This assessment must be ongoing and will change as the adolescent chooses to share more of herself with the social worker.

For social workers with the luxury of meeting with the adolescent on an ongoing basis (such as a prenatal clinic), the focus of the first session may be a brief assessment, attempting to engage the adolescent, setting the stage for trust and giving the teen the opportunity to feel she is being heard. Overlooking the importance of engagement is not only a disservice to the teen but also will adversely affect the chances of an accurate assessment. Thus, by beginning with nonthreatening questions, by appropriately using humor and most importantly by maintaining a non-judgmental attitude, the likelihood of a more thorough assessment will be increased and the stage will be set for future interventions.

CLINICAL CASE MANAGEMENT

Given the consequences of early childbearing and the multifaceted factors contributing to a more positive biopsychosocial outcome, it would be beneficial for the social worker to assume the role of the clinical case manager, coordinating the diverse services that increase the chance for a positive outcome. By completing an accurate and comprehensive assessment, the social worker identifies the needs of each individual adolescent and formulates a comprehensive plan linking the adolescent with appropriate available resources. This may involve educational referrals, referrals to supplemental food programs, group services and/or innovative programs in the community. Thus, the perinatal social worker must be familiar with community resources and network with staff in these programs.

In addition to competent assessment skills and intimate knowledge of community resources, the social worker must value and promote good interdisciplinary collaboration. No discipline can act in a vacuum given the inter-relatedness of the biopsychosocial needs of the childbearing adolescent. Not only should there be ongoing communication but also there should be a structured forum such as monthly meetings with representatives of the various disciplines involved in the care of the population of pregnant adolescents served by the agency. This forum would facilitate communication concerning individual teens, allow for the opportunity to address issues relating to the population served and increase the likelihood of coordinated clinical care.

MOBILIZING THE FAMILY

Support from a parent or guardian can enhance the pregnant adolescent's coping ability and her chances to overcome disadvantages. Therefore, it is important that every attempt be made to include family (ideally with the adolescent's permission) in social work intervention. Pregnancy can disrupt the family system and create conflict or exacerbate a history of conflict. In addition to helping the adolescent inform her parent(s) or guardian of the pregnancy, a social worker may need to assist the family in postpartum planning (i.e., who the primary caregiver will be, the degree of family support, the responsibilities of the teen and educational and daycare arrangements) or may be called for crisis intervention with an adolescent who is leaving home.

Initially, the adolescent's mother (or guardian) and family are likely to be disappointed and angry about the teen's pregnancy and decision to keep and raise the baby. If the mother was a teen mother herself, as a significant number were (Kahn & Anderson: 1992), she may reflect back to limitations caused by her own early childbearing. The adolescent's mother may be nearing a time when her own children would become independent and may be reluctant to become the primary caregiver for this baby. The teen's mother or guardian may regard the teen's pregnancy as a selfish and irresponsible act. Worrying that supporting the teen might condone the pregnancy, while not supporting her may cause pain and suffering, the mother is faced with a difficult decision. If there was conflict in the relationship prior to the pregnancy, the guardian's response may be more drastic. Given the importance of the family's influence on the adolescent's coping and parenting skills, every effort should be made to include the family in the treatment plan. However, this is not always possible and, for some adolescents, may not be beneficial. It is the social worker's task to assess the appropriateness and extent of social work intervention with the family.

INCLUSION OF THE BABY'S FATHER

Clinicians should not underestimate the importance of the "adolescent" father, who may or may not be an adolescent. Even though the importance of the father's inclusion has been well documented (Thompson & Pebbles-Wilkins: 1992, Robinson: 1988, Hardy, Duggen, Masnyk, & Pearson: 1989, Sander & Rosen: 1987), he is far too often overlooked in practice. Clearly, there are fathers who abandon adolescent mothers; however, there are also fathers who have a strong desire to be involved with their child. Not only may the father be living away from the teen mother, but the teen mother may also threaten to withhold the baby from him. To many fathers, this sense of helplessness and vulnerability may be both frustrating and infuriating. Similar social work services that are offered to adolescent mothers must be offered to young fathers if they are to overcome the many barriers to their involvement in their baby's life.

ENHANCING SOCIAL WORK INVOLVEMENT

When working with childbearing teens, it is essential that the perinatal social worker be encouraged to be both innovative and creative. While the staggering caseloads of many social workers may act as a deterrent for such practices, the innovative use of groups, teen mentors and volunteers will be well worth the additional efforts.

Pregnant adolescents, similar to other adolescents, may have heightened needs for peer acceptance yet may feel isolated from their non-pregnant peers. Confused by changing relationships and frightened of both parenting, labor and delivery, they may have major knowledge deficits in these areas. For many of these adolescents, support and/or educational groups may be the modality of choice. In addition, group services to parents, guardians, boyfriends (or husbands) and siblings can enhance an agency's services and increase the likelihood of a positive outcome.

Parenting teens can be utilized as teen mentors to pregnant teens (e.g., parenting teens who are successfully breastfeeding can participate in breastfeeding classes). Again, given the strong influence of peers during the teen years, these mentors can be very successful at imparting information. In addition, the pregnant teen might feel that the parenting teen "really understands." The teen mentor, placed in this "expert" role, can also gain a greater sense of competency and may benefit from the mentoring.

The use of properly trained and supervised volunteers, who have time, energy and motivation, can be an asset to the perinatal social worker. This untapped resource should not be overlooked as volunteers can assist in groups, waiting room programs and outreach efforts and act as friendly visitors on the postpartum floors.

AFTER THE BIRTH OF A HEALTHY BABY

Volumes could be written on social work with adolescent mothers and their children. By the time the baby is born, the adolescent may have negotiated roles and relationships within the family and may be relishing the attention brought by her baby. For many adolescents, the reality of being a young mother becomes clear when the baby is about six months old. The tasks of mothering may be much more difficult than she anticipated and incompatible with her own adolescent needs. The baby may not meet her expectations. There may be conflict with her own guardian over who is the "mommy." There may be changes in her relationship with the father. For these reasons, and as part of the social worker's efforts in coordinating care, there should be strong linkages to adolescent parenting programs. These programs include well baby care, social work services, parenting classes and family planning services.

AFTER THE BIRTH OF A PRETERM OR SICK NEWBORN

Adolescents who find themselves with a sick baby or a baby on the infant's unit or the NICU may not have the luxury of experiencing the "honeymoon period" during the infant's first months of life. These adolescents, their coping abilities clearly tested by early pregnancy and early childbearing, now must manage the care of a sick child, possibly even a chronically sick child.

At best, their child's hospitalization can be a productive encounter for adolescent parents that assists their own developmental and maturational needs and enhances bonding with and learning about their child. At worst, the infant's hospitalization is the latest unfolding of a teenager's troubled, even tragic, life, with massive social pathology already being shifted to a new vulnerable infant.

Again, as pregnancy at an early age may be symptomatic of a chaotic, resource poor, high risk lifestyle, poor pregnancy outcome resulting in the infant's hospitalization may be due to similar variables. For example, a drug-affected infant, a child who fails to thrive because his impoverished parents dilute the formula or a medical condition caused or exacerbated by symptoms that were ignored by an inexperienced, distracted young parent. Maternal substance abuse during pregnancy may result in the birth of a premature or sick infant who may require prolonged hospitalization. Young parents too poor or inexperienced to properly nourish or care for the infant may find the baby does not thrive and requires hospitalization after delivery.

Typically adolescents, especially early and middle adolescents, lack fully developed problem-solving skills, including the ability to plan, and may be intolerant of demands of others (Kriepe: 1983). This may be manifested in lack of visitation and not comprehending why their presence is being requested. An adolescent parent may not yet be capable of understanding her infant's needs, nor her own capabilities to meet those needs (Sadler & Catrone: 1983).

Erikson and others have presented the challenges facing adolescents on their individual paths to maturity. According to Erikson, the overall goal of this stage of life is that of securing an identity (Erikson: 1963). This task will be a gradual one, and not be completed until late adolescence, usually 17 or older. As this sense of self develops, so do higher cognitive processes such as abstract thinking. If this stage comes to a full realization, the adolescent will consolidate a personality that has warmth, empathy and a relatively consolidated sense of self (Buckholz & Gol: 1986). However, the adolescent parent is not necessarily at this relatively late stage of psychosocial development. Therefore, staff is likely to encounter young parents who are ambivalent about their new roles, impulsive and angry at the hospital staff as authority figures (Sadler & Catrone: 1983).

When working with the teen parent of a hospitalized infant, the goals for social work relate to the parents' developmental needs. The social worker must again thoroughly assess the adolescent's developmental strengths and needs in order to support the teen and appropriately plan for the infant's discharge. In the brief time available, the social worker must try to further her coping skills, development and socialization.

Although they may be inconsistent, many teenagers are excellent at techniques of caregiving, from bathing and changing to more difficult problems such as gastrostomy care. This skill can often provide a positive opening for interventions. Giving positive reinforcement on competencies can help the adolescent's self-esteem and promote confidence in handling new situations. Coupling this praise with simple educational statements can be useful. If conflict erupts during a child's hospitalization, this, troubling as it is, can be a learning source for parents, for disagreement can be modeled and goals established.

The specific strengths of each adolescent parent, regardless of how basic they are, need to be continually reinforced. They need to feel more effective in order to better care for their children.

CONCLUSION

It is essential that perinatal social workers working with pregnant and parenting adolescents have a firm understanding of adolescent development and to remember that, while these teens are struggling to accomplish the many tasks of parenting, they are first and foremost adolescents. Being pregnant and a parent during the adolescent years poses many challenges. It is the social worker's role not only to identify the adolescent's limitations but also to identify, support and enhance the adolescent's strengths.

Certainly, there are tremendous disadvantages to early childbearing and there are adolescents who do not succeed. Large case loads and tragic life stories can weaken a social worker's resolve to make a difference. However, positive parenting begins in utero. Hospital social workers working with childbearing adolescents have the opportunity to facilitate the development of competent, self-assured parents.

Accepted for Publication: 05/15/96

REFERENCES

Abrahamse, A.F., Morrison, P.A., and Waite, L.J. (1988) "Teenagers Willing to Consider Single Parenthood: Who Is at Greatest Risk?" *Family Planning Perspectives*, 20(1) 13-18.

Alan Guttmacher Institute (1988) *Facts in Brief.*

Barr, L., and Monserrat, C. (1992) *Working with Pregnant and Parenting Teens.* New Mexico: New Futures Inc.

Brown, S.S. (1988) *Parental Care: Reaching Mothers, Reaching Infants.* Washington, D.C.: National Academy Press.

Buchholz, E.S., and Gol, B. (1986) "More Than Playing House: A Developmental Perspective on the Strengths in Teenage Motherhood." *American Journal of Orthopsychiatry*, 56(3) 347-359.

Burt, M. (1986) "Estimating the Public Costs of Teenage Childbearing." *Family Planning Perspectives*, 18(5) 221-226.

Child Welfare League of America (1995) *Adolescent Childbearing in the United States.*

Children's Defense Fund (1986) "The Broadeer Challenge of Teen Pregnancy Prevention." *Children's Defense Fund Reports*, 8: 1, 6, and 8.

Dash, L. (1989) *When Children Want Children.* New York: Penguin Books (p. 10).

Elkind, D. (1988) *The Hurried Child.* Massachusetts: Addison-Wesley Publishing Company.

Erikson, E. (1963) *Childhood and Society.* New York: W.W. Norton Co.

The Facts: Adolescent Sexuality, Pregnancy and Parenthood. (1991) Washington, D.C.: Center for Population Options.

Fraser, A.M., Brockert, J.E., and Ward, R.H. (1995) "Association of Young Maternal Age with Adverse Reproductive Outcomes." *The New England Journal of Medicine,* 17(332) 113-117.

Furstenberg, F.F., Brooks-Gunn, J., and Morgan, S.P. (1987) *Adolescent Mothers and Their Children in Later Life.* Cambridge, U.K.: Cambridge University Press.

Hall, G.S. (1904) *Adolescence.* New York: Appleton.

Hamburg, B. (1986) "Subsets of Adolescent Mothers: Developmental, Biomedical, and Psychological Issues." In Lancaster, J.B., and Hamburg, B. (eds.) *School-Age Pregnancy and Parenthood: Biosocial Dimensions.* New York: Aldine DeGruyter (pp. 117-146).

Hardy, J.B., Duggen, A.K., Masnyk, K., and Pearson, C. (1989) "Fathers of Children Born to Young Urban Mothers." *Family Planning Perspectives,* 21(4) 159-164.

Hayes, C.D. ed., (1987) *Risking the Future: Adolescent Sexuality, Pregnancy and Childbearing,* Vol. 1. Washington, D.C.: National Academy Press.

Jones, E.F. (1986) *Teenage Pregnancy in Industrialized Countries.* New Haven: Yale University Press.

Jorgenson, S.R. (1983) "Sex Education and the Reduction of Adolescent Pregnancy: Prospects for the 1980's." *Journal of Early Adolescence,* 3, 38-52.

Kahn, J.R., and Anderson, K.E. (1992) "Intergeneral Patterns of Teenage Fertility." *Demography.*

Kriepe, R. (1983) "Prevention of Adolescent Pregnancy, a Developmental Approach" in McAnarney, E. *Premature Adolescent and Parenthood.* New York: Grune and Stratton (pp. 37-60).

Leland, M. (1987). "The Role of Congress in Risking the Future: A Symposium on the National Academy of Sciences Report on Teenage Pregnancy." *Family Planning Perspectives,* 19(3) 121-122.

Lockhart, L.L., and Wodarski, J.S. (1990) "Teenage Pregnancy: Implications for Social Work Practice." *Family Therapy,* 17(1) 29-47.

Makinson, C. (1985) "The Health Consequences of Teenage Fertility." *Family Planning Perspectives,* 17(3) 132-139.

Mercer, R.T., Hackley, K.C., and Bostrom, A. (1984) "Adolescent Motherhood: Comparison of Outcomes with Older Mothers." *Journal of Adolescent Health Care,* 5(1) 7-13.

National Association of Social Workers (1987) *Encyclopedia of Social Work,* (18th ed.). Silver Spring, MD, 5(1) 7-13.

Nichols, F. (1991) "Secondary Prevention with the Pregnant Adolescent." In Humenick, S.S., Wilkerson, N.N., and Paul, N.W. (eds.) *Adolescent Pregnan-*

cy: Nursing Perspectives on Prevention. New York: March of Dimes Foundation (pp. 33-43).

Piaget, J. (1972) "Intellectual Evolution from Adolescence to Adulthood." *Human Development,* 15, 1-12.

Rich, O.J. (1991) "Family Focused Tertiary Prevention with the Adolescent Mother and Her Child." In Humenick, S.S., Wilkerson, N.N., and Paul, N.W. (eds.) *Adolescent Pregnancy: Nursing Perspectives on Prevention.* New York: March of Dimes Foundation (pp. 137-154).

Robinson, B. (1988) *Teenage Fathers.* Massachusetts: Lexington Books.

Sadler, L.S., and Catrone, C. (1983) "The Adolescent Parent: A Dual Developmental Crisis." *Journal of Adolescent Health Care,* 5(3).

Sander, J.H., and Rosen, J.L. (1987) "Teenage Fathers: Working with the Neglected Partner in Adolescent Childbearing." *Family Planning Perspectives,* 19(3) 107-110.

Scholl, T.O., Decker, E., Karp, R.J., Greene, G., and DeSales, M. (1984) "Early Adolescent Pregnancy: A Comparative Study of Pregnancy Outcome in Young Adolescents and Mature Women." *Journal of Adolescent Health Care,* 5, 167-171.

Thompson, M.S., and Peebles-Wilkens, W. (1992) "The Impact of Formal, Informal, and Societal Support Networks on the Psychological Well-Being of Black Adolescent Mothers." *Social Work,* 37(4) 323-328.

Young, C.L., McMahon, J., Bowman, V.M., and Thompson, D. (1989) "Adolescent Third-Trimester Enrollment in Prenatal Care." *Journal of Adolescent Health Care,* 5(3).

Zabin, L.S., and Hayward, S.C. (1993) *Adolescent Sexual Behavior and Childbearing.* London: Sage Publications.

Postpartum Depression:
A Review for Perinatal Social Workers

Virginia N. Walther, MSW

SUMMARY. Postpartum depression is a common and treatable clinical syndrome which effects up to fifty percent of all women and which can best be considered as a triad of disorders. Postpartum blues, postpartum affective disorders or major depressions, and postpartum psychosis have distinct symptoms with corresponding implications for social work interventions and treatment strategies. The role of prevention can be pivotal in terms of reducing negative impacts of psychological problems after birth and minimizing adverse consequences for the new baby and all family members. *[Article copies available for a fee from The Haworth Document Delivery Service: 1-800-342-9678. E-mail address: getinfo@haworth.com]*

Postpartum depression is a common and treatable clinical syndrome which illustrates the spectrum from "normal" changes to pathological phenomena which may occur in women following delivery.

Postpartum psychological reactions have been described since fourth century B.C. Hippocrates considered postpartum depression to be a specific disease. He speculated that misdirected milk was carried toward the mother's head causing cerebral engorgement and the resultant symptoms of agitation, delirium and mania. It is now commonly accepted that clinical depression in predisposed individuals can be precipitated by stress; and

---

Virginia N. Walther is Senior Assistant Director, Department of Social Work Services, The Mount Sinai Hospital, 1 Gustave L. Levy Place, Box 1252, New York, NY 10029.

[Haworth co-indexing entry note]: "Postpartum Depression: A Review for Perinatal Social Workers." Walther, Virginia N. Co-published simultaneously in *Social Work in Health Care* (The Haworth Press, Inc.) Vol. 24, No. 3/4, 1997, pp. 99-111; and: *Fundamentals of Perinatal Social Work: A Guide for Clinical Practice with Women, Infants, and Families* (ed: Regina Furlong Lind, and Debra Honig Bachman) The Haworth Press, Inc., 1997, pp. 99-111. Single or multiple copies of this article are available for a fee from The Haworth Document Delivery Service [1-800-342-9678, 9:00 a.m. - 5:00 p.m. (EST). E-mail address: getinfo@haworth.com].

the postpartum period, often described as a maturational crisis involving identity reformation, endocrine changes and role transition, can exert such stress upon the new mother. However, the usefulness of this knowledge and our understanding of postpartum depression remains limited.

Authors such as Barbara Kaplan believe that we know little about postpartum depression largely because we know little about the larger prevalence of depression among all pregnant women. Kaplan suggests that Western culture maintains an attitude of pluralistic ignorance towards depression during pregnancy. "It would be very helpful to have carefully collected information about the emotional course of pregnancy, so that if the myth of the joyful, placid pregnant woman is inaccurate, it might be replaced by a more realistic image" (Kaplan, 1986). There is undoubtedly confusion between what is the normal course of pregnancy and what is a depressive disorder occurring during the course of pregnancy or postpartum.

Several methodological issues in the research of postpartum depression have contributed to the lack of consensus in defining and understanding the phenomenon of postpartum depression. These include a poor understanding of the psychological correlates of hormonal changes. Because hormonal shifts are so marked during and after pregnancy, researchers sought to establish a clear, causal link between postpartum hormonal changes and depression. This theory of a specific hormonal etiology has been largely unsubstantiated as the majority of women who experience equal hormonal changes do not become clinically depressed after birth. Research has also been marred by a lack of uniformity in the definition of the postpartum period and variations in the operational definitions of postpartum depression and its psychological characteristics. The terms postpartum depression, postpartum psychosis and postpartum blues have been used interchangeably without differentiation. Furthermore, many studies have tended to use retrospective and concurrent reports to evaluate predictive relationships instead of using prospective studies to attempt to predict who will become depressed (Gise, 1984).

In spite of the controversies surrounding the definition, etiology and treatment of postpartum depression, for social workers in perinatal settings, the diagnosis presents an issue of importance for both clinical treatment interventions as well as primary prevention and care. Although largely undetected and untreated by medical and psychiatric providers, postpartum depression is a common phenomenon, affecting ten to twenty percent of all women within three months after childbirth. While among the most treatable psychiatric diagnoses, it is estimated that only twenty percent of those who are afflicted actually receive mental health treatment.

Most remain either undiagnosed or improperly diagnosed. The Diagnostic and Statistical Manual of Mental Disorders (American Psychiatric Association, 1994) still does not have a category for psychiatric disorders of the puerperium period. Characterized by depressed feelings, anxiety, stress, low self-esteem and marital instability, postpartum depression probably is the result of an interplay between biomedical, psychological and social factors. All individual family members and their new as well as longstanding relationships with one another can be significantly and adversely affected by the disorder. Hamilton stresses the need for treatment within the context of the new-mother role (Hamilton, 1962). Social workers, who bring an understanding and appreciation of the postnatal context for women and their families, are often positioned to offer early interventions which are specific to this transitional stage of life as well as to offer psycho education programs during the prenatal period focused on prevention of maternal emotional disorders.

IMPACT OF POSTPARTUM DEPRESSION ON FAMILIES

It is estimated that in the general population depression is almost twice as prevalent among women as among men. About five percent of the female population will experience depression at some point in the life cycle with the reproductive years being the time of highest risk for the development of a depressive episode. There is also research evidence pointing to an increased incidence of emotional disorders during the period of childbearing and lactation. Postpartum depression has generally been defined as occurring up to one year following childbirth (Gise, 1984). Severe sleep disturbance and anxiety may be predictors of depression although many women give a normal outward appearance when depressed. Although postpartum depression is rarely diagnosed by obstetrical providers of care and symptoms are hidden or misdiagnosed, it has adverse effects on many families with new babies (Hopkins et al., 1984; Gruen, 1990). Pitt, in reviewing the literature on the incidence of mild to moderate depressive episodes among women after childbirth, reported a range of 3 percent to thirty-one percent depending on the criteria used for diagnosis (Pitt, 1982). The postpartum period may be justifiably characterized as a developmental crisis in the life of a woman accompanied by transitional changes in roles and relationships as well as considerable emotional upheaval. Social pressures on parents to idealize new parenthood and to diminish any negative feelings such as fear, anxiety, exhaustion and ambivalence contribute to the stresses experienced by a parent in transition (Gruen, 1990). Both practitioners and researchers agree that a large proportion of women experience a range of emotional reactions generally characterized as depressive in nature and occurring as a response to physical, social and psychological changes associated with birth. These responses during the postpartum period do not constitute a single syndrome but rather are usually grouped according to onset, intensity and duration.

A number of authors have proposed a tripartite classification scheme for the spectrum of postpartum emotional disorders (Inwood, 1985; Gise, 1984), which are:

- Postpartum Blues or adjustment disorder with depressed mood
- Postpartum Depression or major affective disorder
- Postpartum psychosis or psychotic depression of the puerperal period

While research on postpartum depression varies in definitions and methodologies and even reveals contradictory findings at times, most agree with this delineation of three levels of the disorder.

POSTPARTUM ADJUSTMENT DISORDERS

Postpartum blues may be defined as mild mood disorders which are transient situational disturbances or adjustment disorders which are fleeting, benign and prevalent enough to be considered normal. These mild disturbances may also occur during pregnancy as well. Adjustment disorders involve maladaptive reactions that either interfere with social or occupational functioning, or are in excess of a woman's baseline emotional status, and usually occur within three months of stressful experiences—in this case, childbirth. Postpartum blues may be a prelude to postpartum depression in some cases. The "baby blues" are estimated to occur in up to fifty percent of postpartum women with symptoms peaking around the fifty postpartum day independent of breast-feeding or length of stay in the hospital (Kendall, 1985). Dysphoric symptoms including tearfulness, anxiety, feelings of emotional lability and fatigue may last for several days but are generally self limiting, and usually last no longer than two weeks. Women may express concern with somatic complaints such as headaches and sleep disturbance, experience low self esteem, voice negative feelings about marital relationships and harbor negative or ambivalent feelings about the new infant as well as older children. Feelings toward the newborn may show considerable variation with some women expressing distress over what they perceive as lack of maternal feelings or bonding within the first few days after delivery. Interestingly, studies in Europe, Asia and Africa lend cross-cultural validation to the widespread nature of these experiences among new mothers. However, in cultures in which women have little marital, family or social supports in assuming their new roles, stressors may be exacerbated.

Psychodynamics posed for postpartum adjustment disorders include unrealistically high and idealized expectations about the rewards and joys of new motherhood which can result in perceived or actual failure in the parental role and resultant lowered self-esteem and disappointments. Women may also experience a feeling of depletion and loss of the pregnant state and a sense of oneness with the baby. Finally, many new mothers experience the postpartum period as a transitional crisis with accompanying ambivalence about assuming the tasks and responsibilities of motherhood. Indeed, well established coping mechanisms may not suffice although new ones have not yet been developed, and a child's unpredictable behaviors and demands can prove overwhelming.

MAJOR DEPRESSION

According to the DSM-III-R, major postpartum depression is characterized by a depressed mood or anhedonia which must be present for at least two weeks. The lay interpretation of depression focuses on the presence of sadness but the clinical diagnosis of a major depressive episode depends on a combination of symptoms, that is a syndrome, which necessitates that three or four of the following be present:

- Change in weight
- Sleep disturbance
- Psychomotor agitation or retardation
- Fatigue
- Feelings of worthlessness or excessive guilt
- Diminished concentration or indecisiveness
- Recurrent thoughts of death or suicidal ideation

The incidence of major postpartum depression is ten to twenty percent, and the recurrence rate with subsequent pregnancies is twenty to thirty percent. The clinical course of a major depression may begin within days of delivery or may become manifest up to one year postpartum, lasting six weeks or longer. Because symptoms may not emerge until weeks following delivery and because symptoms may not be apparent unless specific inquiry is made, many postpartum depressions remain unheeded and untreated. Most investigators suggest that postpartum depression results from a complex interplay between the physiological and psychological stresses of the peripartum period; adjustments to child care responsibilities and new role demands; inadequate social supports; and a psychological or biological vulnerability to depression. While the etiology of the diagnosis is multifaceted, psychodynamic theories of postpartum depression include:

1. Unresolved dynamics in conflictual family relationships.
2. A neglectful or abusive relationship with one's own mother which results in an inadequate role model with accompanying identity confusion and rejection of the maternal role. The infant's cries for help may be experienced ambivalently as a call for help or as an angry rejection of the insecure parent.
3. Unfulfilled dependency needs resulting in an inability to attend to the newborn's needs.

A postpartum major depression can carry considerable morbidity to the mother, child and family. Emotionally hungry, the depressed mother is first and foremost preoccupied with herself and not her infant. As a consequence, she may fail to establish the gratifying experience of mutuality, imitation of vocalizations, movements and expressions that bring mother and child so closely and delightfully together. Ambivalent attachments can set a tone of an impersonal relationship and its intrapsychic trappings throughout the child's life.

POSTPARTUM PSYCHOSIS

Postpartum psychosis is generally classified as a separate disorder from postpartum depression and is characterized by psychosis, suicidal or homicidal ideation. The incidence of postpartum psychosis is said to be one to two per 1,000 live births. The disorder is of the severity often to warrant psychiatric hospitalization and careful monitoring but may also be treated on an outpatient or partial hospitalization basis. The onset of postpartum psychosis occurs within six weeks of delivery with the highest incidence within the first three weeks following delivery. Prodromal symptoms of irritability, crying and insomnia are common. A flamboyant, acute and manic picture may occur soon after delivery and, in fact, signals a good prognosis. Dramatic symptoms include excitement, restlessness and pressured speech. Rapid changes to a depressed state may occur and be associated with disorientation, irritability, restlessness and visual hallucinations. Delusional material will usually incorporate elements of the childbirth experience; e.g., someone swapped babies or the devil was the baby's father. Delusional material may also involve the idea that the baby is dead (Gise, 1984; Kendall, 1985), and suicidal and infanticidal ideation has been reported. Because of the real risk of destructive acts towards herself or her baby, the mother's symptoms must be carefully managed and supervised.

Postpartum psychosis has often been described as an organic-like psychosis caused by dramatic fluctuations in hormones. While this explanation has always been intriguing for its biological obviousness, it has never been prospectively validated. This leads to the potential for research flaws in an attempt to simplistically and directly correlate interactions between life events and measurable alterations in hormones; in other words, to find a reductionist biological explanation for a very complex bio-psychosocial phenomenon.

In summary, there will continue to be difficulty making diagnostic assessments of postpartum depression as long as many of the normal symptoms of pregnancy mimic depression. As a part of the normal gestational course, many pregnant women experience weight change, fatigue, psychomotor retardation, mood liability, increased somatic concern, anxiety in anticipation of their new roles and responsibilities, etc. Because the normal emotional paths of pregnancy are not well researched nor is depression during pregnancy understood in terms of its prevalence, physical symptoms and psychological disorders can be confused. What is clear is that postpartum depression is the result of the interplay between endocrinological, biochemical, neurophysiological, genetic, psychological, social, cultural and sleep-related variables among others. Barbara Kaplan writes,

> It is important to remember that pregnancy is a complex biological process occurring in a significant psychosocial context. Any interpretation of mood change . . . has to consider that pregnancy brings about many physiological changes, occurs in a social context and that any circumstances surrounding the pregnancy occur together with and in relation to this major biological event. It is thus an excellent example of a psychobiological interaction. (Kaplan, 1986)

PSYCHOSOCIAL FACTORS AS CONTRIBUTING
TO POSTPARTUM DEPRESSION

There have been numerous factors suggested as playing a role in the development and experience of postpartum depression. Authors such as Melges examined maternal conflicts about assuming the role of mother. Parenting a noncommunicative infant was speculated as a hindrance to self-definition since there is little interpersonal feedback and less distinction between self and other in early maternal-child relationships. Melges particularly postulated that although these women were committed to being mothers, they had rejected their own mothers as role models for imitation and identification but had nothing to substitute for such an absence. Thus, they had fragile identities as parents and had few maps for new behaviors in the maternal role. When coupled with poor marital or other social supports, or when exacerbated by other stressful social circumstances such as sleep deprivation, the postpartum woman is at risk for depression. Women whose own mothers had been rejecting or neglectful might indeed begin to mimic these learned behaviors (Melges, 1968).

Some authors delve into situational factors such as family death or job loss, that have placed significant stress on vulnerable new mothers. Such stressors in combination with the birth may provoke anxiety, feelings of loss, and depression during the postpartum period. Chronic strains such as marital discord and conflict, unrealistic expectations for the rewards of parenthood, past histories of depression, and physical illness, may also be related to the etiology of postpartum depression. Again, social pressures on new parents to acknowledge only the joys and positive aspects of new parenthood contribute to the possibility of despair when parents reveal experiences with anger, fear and other negative feelings which in turn are minimized or denied by others. As Gruen states, "Depression in response to death, divorce, or job loss is culturally acceptable, whereas depression in response to the arrival of a child is not culturally approved" (Gruen, 1990). The very real losses associated with new parenthood such as loss of independence or identity remain unrecognized and often become internalized as failures in the new role with the accompanying feelings of depression. Researchers have examined the impact of social support systems in mitigating postpartum depression. Kaplan (1986) considers that people experiencing major upheavals in their lives are more susceptible to the influence of others than they are at times of normal functioning and that the quality of support offered by others may have the effect of loading the dice in favor of a good or poor outcome. We do know, however, that depressed individuals can become interpersonally aversive to family and friends and are characterized by poor social skills even when support systems are in place.

Cognitive theories of postpartum depression have focused on the preexisting personality characteristics of a new mother that predispose her to depression and which magnify the likelihood that she will harbor unrealistic ideas of childbirth and the maternal role. As former coping mechanisms do not work in the new role, mothers experience a sense of failure, lowered self-esteem and bewilderment about how to cope with a new situation. New behaviors must be learned in order to restore feelings of competence and a positive self image.

As previously stated, not one of these theories alone provides a simple etiologic explanation for postpartum depression, yet each shed some light about variables in combination with biological factors which contribute to its causation and to the experience of women suffering from the diagnosis.

TREATMENT FOR POSTPARTUM BLUES

As hospital lengths of stay are being reduced to as brief a period as twenty-four hours following uncomplicated deliveries in some states, social workers on hospital Obstetrics services may not be in a position to detect the beginnings of a postpartum depression whose symptoms will generally not become manifest until about three days to one week post delivery. Therefore, the four-to-six-week postpartum visit may be the ideal time to assess women for depression; and the first well baby appointment should not be a missed opportunity for assessment as well. For women suffering from the postpartum blues, ego supportive interventions may be an optimum approach to treatment. Acknowledgment of the realistic frustrations and difficulties involved in caring for an infant and mastering the role transition to new parenthood combined with constructive suggestions for managing these inherent stressors may be pivotal to women, especially to those with few social support or positive role models. Support groups are increasingly being offered to new parents both as a skills building forum as well as a socialization experience with a positive reference group with common interests. With the more widespread recognition of the commonplace nature of postpartum blues, community-based support mutual aid networks for new mothers who are depressed are developing such as National Depression After Delivery, a self-help organization which puts new mothers in touch with support groups, literature and peer telephone assistance, among other services. The advantage of group interventions is that the group validates the experiences and stresses of motherhood and permits the expression of the common, yet complex ambivalent feelings in a nonjudgmental milieu where one can also receive acceptance, aid and advice. The validation and acceptance of depressed feelings, in and of itself, is powerful in reducing individual members' feelings of isolation and personal deficiency. A new network of social relationships in which members share interests and concerns and in which individuals receive recognition of their strengths and abilities is a forum in which problem solving can likely occur and new coping capacities emerge. These groups are truly self-help in substance and in spirit.

Social workers may also be pivotal in helping to enlist family members to assume a more hands-on helping role for the new mother and to support her during this critical time of adjustment. Psycho education as a treatment approach for both mother and key family members is also helpful in normalizing and educating them about the experiences of postpartum depression and engaging them in concerted coping strategies that are family focused. As family members develop empathy and understanding for this diagnosis and they develop ways to appropriately respond and assist the new mother, she often will feel less isolated and inadequate.

TREATMENT FOR MAJOR POSTPARTUM DEPRESSION

The treatment for a major postpartum depression may include:

- Antidepressant medication
- Psychotherapy
- Extra support, particularly with child care responsibilities

All interventions with women suffering a major depression should include an assessment of the potential for child abuse or neglect, and the woman's fears about harming the baby must be assessed and monitored carefully. Outside of these special considerations related to the newborn, the treatment of postpartum depression is similar to that involved with other depressive disorders occurring at other times. While psychopharmacological interventions are generally recommended, these should be offered in conjunction with psychosocial interventions based on the individual's social context and psychological baseline. Work with family members and a woman's larger community network should also focus on developing support which can lighten the burden of new child care responsibilities during this demanding period, especially in light of the fact that much research demonstrates the relationship between depression and low levels of social support from family members. Referrals to appropriate community resources can be an important role for social workers in terms of broadening available supports both of an emotional and practical nature, which may act as a buffer against the strains of stressful life events.

Many women experience relief from seeing a social worker or other mental health professional in psychotherapeutic counseling who is both empathetic and knowledgeable about the disorder. Psychotherapy is recommended when support, information and acceptance of the depression is not adequate to relieve symptoms and when counseling related to underlying conflicts is indicated. Again, support groups are another valuable resource for women suffering from postpartum depression. The communion with other new mothers who are also experiencing depression or who have "been there" and recovered is therapeutic in the validation of the reality of the condition and the alleviation of the isolation associated with it.

TREATMENT OF POSTPARTUM PSYCHOSIS

The treatment of postpartum psychosis should be managed by or in conjunction with a psychiatrist and may be carried out on an inpatient or ambulatory basis or in a day hospital. The health care professional and the family should be alert to potential destructive acts to the woman herself or to her infant. Adequate monitoring and supervision are critical (Gise, 1984). Treatment in addition to anti-depressant medication may consist of psychotherapy, support, reinforcement of the patient's abilities to function as a mother, and at times, somatic intervention such as electroconvulsive therapy. Psychiatric units in which mothers and babies may be hospitalized together, while rare, are effective in promoting maternal-child bonding as well as providing psychiatric interventions.

THE ROLE OF PREVENTION

The treatment of postpartum depression can be greatly enhanced by an ounce of prevention. With multifactorial causation, reducing any of the contributing factors may lessen the likelihood that a serious psychological problem will develop following birth. New prospective studies have suggested that rates of depression during pregnancy are similar to those developed and diagnosed after pregnancy. Furthermore, prenatal depression has been found to be a predictor of postpartum depression. Therefore, in both the prenatal setting and during postpartum hospital stays, patients should be referred to social workers when sources of stress for a patient become apparent. The incidence of postpartum depression may be reduced or may benefit from early interventions including psycho education; parenting education and support; community resource referrals; psychotherapy of an individual, family or groups nature; and reassurance. When maternal anxiety and depression are reduced, newborns are also protected from the consequences of maternal deprivation which accompany postpartum depression.

Therefore, attempts during the prenatal period to identify women at high risk for postpartum depression are key. For example, women who appear excessively anxious, who have a history of past depressions, who are having marital or family problems or who have experienced other stressful life events should be referred for evaluation and early intervention planning. In addition, educating women in childbirth education classes or other antenatal forums about the real risk factors and early symptoms associated with postpartum depression and those resources available to help them cope with such an occurrence, can facilitate their ability to access appropriate preventive and early mental health care interventions.

Postpartum depression and its consequences for entire families pose an important challenge to social workers. The prenatal period, the postpartum hospitalization, the two-week well baby appointment, and the postpartum visit should be utilized to assess women for early signs and symptoms of depression. At one urban medical center, perinatal social workers, together with the division of liaison psychiatry, have begun to use the Edinburgh Postnatal Depression Scale (EPDS) to screen women for depression. This scale was developed specifically to detect postpartum depression and was shown to be valid and reliable in large community surveys in the United Kingdom (Cox et al., 1987). Because cultural factors and attitudes towards postpartum depression differ in the United States, this scale should be retested for validity and reliability prior to advocating its widespread use. Other screening tools may similarly be developed by providers which are culturally and socially syntonic with the population being served. Such tools may be economical, easy for patients to self-administer and also easily scored. Further screening enables providers to intervene early with a population who have too often been undetected and underserved.

Accepted for Publication: 06/14/96

REFERENCES

American Psychiatric Association (1994). *Diagnostic and Statistical Manual of Mental Disorders IV.* Washington, D.C.: American Psychiatric Association.

Cox, J., Holden, J. & Saqovsk, R. (1987). Detection of Postnatal Depression: Development of the 10-Item Edinburgh Postnatal Scale. *British Journal of Psychiatry*, 150: 782-786.

Gise, L. (1984). Psychiatric Implications of Pregnancy. In Cherry & Merkate (Eds.) *Complications of Pregnancy: Medical, Surgical, Gynecologic, Psychosocial and Perinatal*. Baltimore: Williams and Wilkins, 194-250.

Gruen, D.S. (1990). Postpartum Depression: A Debilitating Yet Often Unassessed Problem. *Health and Social Work*, 262: 261-270.

Hamilton, J.A. (1962). *Postpartum Psychiatric Problems*. St. Louis: CV Mosby.

Hopkins, J. & Marcus, M. (1984). Postpartum Depression: A Critical Review. *Psychological Bulletin*, 95: 498-515.

Inwood, D.G. (1985). *Recent Advances in Postpartum Psychiatric Disorders*. Washington, D.C.: American Psychiatric Press, Inc.

Kaplan, B. (1986). Causes and Attributes of Depression During Pregnancy. *Women and Health*, 8: 23-30.

Kendall, R. (1985). Emotional and Physical Factors in the Genesis of Puerperal Mental Disorders. *Journal of Psychosomatic Research*, 29: 3-11.

Melges, F.T. (1968). *Postpartum Psychiatric Syndromes in Psychosomatic Medicine*. New York: Harper and Row.

Pitt, B. (1982). Depression and Childbirth. In Paykel (Ed.) *Handbook of Affective Disorders*. New York: Guilford Press.

Pugh, T.J., Jerath, B.K., Schmidt, W.M. & Reed, R.B. (1963). Rates of Mental Disease Related to Child Bearing. *New England Journal of Medicine*, 268: 1224-1228.

Parenting a Technology Assisted Infant: Coping with Occupational Stress

Kathleen E. Murphy, PhD, LCSW

SUMMARY. This article presents a brief description of the stress factors which families experience during care at home of technology dependent infants and children. The experience of stress and the coping strategies used by family members is organized in terms of the stages of adaptation to home care over time. In addition, the stress and how families cope with the stress is discussed in light of existing theories regarding occupational stress, especially as it relates to role strain, role captivity and role conflict. *[Article copies available for a fee from The Haworth Document Delivery Service: 1-800-342-9678. E-mail address: getinfo@haworth.com]*

BACKGROUND

God damn the medical profession and God bless them. I wouldn't trade in a minute of the time I've had with my son, and I'd trade it all in a minute.

During the last 30 years, advances in medical technology (e.g., apnea monitors, positive pressure ventilators, phrenic nerve pacers, hemodialysis, and infusion pumps) and the technical skills related to mechanical life support have contributed to the survival of infants and children who formerly would have died as a consequence of extreme prematurity, trauma,

---

Kathleen E. Murphy is a Social Worker in private practice in Glenview, IL.

[Haworth co-indexing entry note]: "Parenting a Technology Assisted Infant: Coping with Occupational Stress." Murphy, Kathleen E. Co-published simultaneously in *Social Work in Health Care* (The Haworth Press, Inc.) Vol. 24, No. 3/4, 1997, pp. 113-126; and: *Fundamentals of Perinatal Social Work: A Guide for Clinical Practice with Women, Infants, and Families* (ed: Regina Furlong Lind, and Debra Honig Bachman) The Haworth Press, Inc., 1997, pp. 113-126. Single or multiple copies of this article are available for a fee from The Haworth Document Delivery Service [1-800-342-9678, 9:00 a.m. - 5:00 p.m. (EST). E-mail address: getinfo@haworth.com].

113

catastrophic illness or other chronic impairment. While improvements in perinatal care, neonatology and neonatal intensive care have reduced neonatal mortality (USDHHS, 1982; Office of Technology Assessment (OTA), 1987), in some instances the physical insufficiency of such children has required long-term or permanent mechanical ventilation and other life support. In the past, because of their technical and medical needs, technology assisted infants and children were routinely confined to neonatal or pediatric intensive care units for years–a necessary placement in an extremely costly environment often to the detriment of the developmental needs of the children (Children's Home Health Network of Illinois Report (CHHNI), 1984). It has only been within the last decade that families have been able to realistically expect to be able to care for their technology assisted child at home.

Long-term dependence on mechanical life support at home is not a new phenomena. There were hundreds of polio survivors living at home in the United States on mechanical support after the epidemics of the '50s (Rehabilitation Institute of Chicago, 1981). Unlike the polio population, however, the current pediatric home care population is a diverse group with a wide range of medical diagnoses, many of which are rare. For some there is the need for multiple technologies and diverse services to be provided in diverse circumstances and environments. Until recently, the size and location of the technology assisted population was largely determined by the location of pediatric teaching hospitals, physician attitudes toward aggressive treatment and parental willingness to pursue aggressive treatment (OTA, 1987). Whatever the impetus, the population of medically fragile, medically complex infants and children has grown significantly and will continue to grow over time (CHHNI, 1987; OTA, 1987). For children and families, care at home is certainly the most appropriate as well as cost effective alternative to hospitalization (Bone, 1987; OTA, 1987).

However, learning how to care for and parent a technology assisted child at home is qualitatively different from the care of a technology dependent adult. Children, especially the tiny infant born prematurely, not only need supervised, quality care; they also require special opportunities for growth and development. Further, an understanding of families' as well as children's needs is critical for care at home to provide for optimal growth and development of potential (Stein and Jessop, 1984).

All children exist in the context of a family and the impact on the family caring for an infant requiring technological support has been the focus of attention in recent years (Hochstadt and Yost, 1991). The fact that technology assisted children can be cared for safely at home rather than in the hospital has been well established. There is little doubt that theoretically it is psychologically and socially better for the child to live at home. However, except for a few studies, little is known about the effect of this type of home care on the family system or on the child's perceptions of his or her life on mechanical support, but what is known relates to the stressful nature of the experience for all family members.

THE STRESS OF DEALING WITH HOME HEALTH NURSES

Who's in charge–that's the big one. Some try to tell you what to do or where our place is in our own home . . . They have a difficult time realizing that they are not the one in charge–I am.

Change, no matter how great or small, creates the opportunity for or the environment of stress. Stress occurs in response to a challenge to existing state of family equilibrium which requires some change from the previous ways of functioning. In the ideal world, "going home" from the NICU or PICU is a much desired goal but in the real world of the medically complex, technology assisted infant, going home creates stress on all of the systems involved.

Through clinical experience and the process of research interviews conducted by the author with families of technology assisted children in Illinois, the primary stress factors identified in home care were found to include: dealing with nurses in the home, the financial burden of home care and the emotional aspects of dealing with having a technology assisted child. While most parents feel they were adequately involved in the discharge planning process and feel they receive adequate training to be able to care for their child at home, a common concern has to do with the lack of preparation they feel they received for the "rest" of home care. Each of the primary stresses (nurses, finances and emotions) affects a variety of aspects of family functioning; however, because there is often the need for extensive nursing care, sometimes even 12 to 18 hours per day, this stressor is a singularly difficult issue for families that is largely unanticipated. In fact, parents are often so affected by the presence of nursing staff in the home that it overwhelms all other issues related to dealing with a child dependent on technology.

Of the numerous problems in dealing with nurses identified by parents, the most recurrent are: conflicts over authority and control (e.g., who's in charge in the home, the nurse or the parent), and judgments made by nurses to family members about the families' lifestyle (e.g., standards of care, discipline of the other children, marital relationships and religious values). The presence of nurses also affects the various relationships within the family. The loss of privacy due to the presence of a non-family member inhibits marital, sibling and parental relationships. Siblings get angry about the nurses' interference in their lives and feel isolated by the nurses from the technology assisted child. Siblings also report that the nurses they like best are those who talked with them and treated them like real people–a rather sad commentary on the siblings' experience of having a brother or sister with special needs.

The presence of nurses affects the scheduling of a variety of aspects of family living as even outings have to be timed to coincide with change of shift and nursing coverage. Parents report not leaving the home when new nurses are on shift and only feeling comfortable leaving a few nurses with total responsibility for the technology assisted child for any extended period of time.

Parents talk about having developed a variety of ways to cope with the stress of nurses in the home including staff meetings, written communications, and organized training and orientation, but not all parents are able to deal with the authority and control issues this directly. Some parents, especially single parents, choose to not address problems with the nurses at all rather than risk "rocking the boat." They also learn fairly quickly that it is important to maintain a "professional" employer/employee relationship with the nurses rather than view them as "friends" of the family. However, this is a difficult lesson, especially since mothers learn to rely on the nurses for emotional support during the anxiety-filled early months of home care.

COPING WITH THE STRESS

According to Menaghan (1983), coping, like the concept of stress, is a generally understood term which encompasses a range of concepts, including coping resources, coping styles and coping efforts. "Coping resources" are generalized attitudes and skills that are used across situations and may include: attitudes about the self, such as self-esteem; attitudes about the world; intellectual skills, such as cognitive flexibility or analytic ability; and interpersonal skills. "Coping styles" are coping strategies which are the typical or preferred way an individual approaches problems, such as: withdrawal vs. involvement; denial vs. confrontation; active vs. reactive and so forth. "Coping efforts" are specific actions, overt or covert, which are utilized in specific situations with the intention of reducing stress (Pearlin and Schooler, 1987; Morris and Engle, 1981; Andrews et al., 1978).

Within the family literature, McCubbin et al. (1981) have identified five factors which they feel serve to mediate how a family reacts to and copes with stress, including: acquiring social support from relatives and friends; reframing and redefining stressful events to make them manageable; spiritual support; acquiring and accepting help from the community; and passive appraisal of problematic issues in order to minimize reactivity. Numerous other authors affirm the importance of social support from within the circle of family and friends as well as the community (Turner, 1983; McCubbin, M., 1984; Gallagher et al., 1983; Kazak, 1986; Stuifbergen, 1987). These same authors also cite certain personality characteristics and general attitudes, such as seeing stress as "challenge" rather than as "burden," as mediators of stress and an influence on the development and use of various coping efforts. A number of research studies and clinical accounts identify specific coping strategies used by families of chronically ill children. These tend to be similar to those identified by McCubbin et al. with one major addition: "information seeking" is reported as the most frequently used coping strategy (Coffman, 1983; Brimblecombe, 1984; Barbarin et al., 1985; Horner et al., 1987). This need for information is consistent with what parents have identified in the clinical accounts on stress in home care (OTA, 1987; Report of Brook Lodge, 1983).

After significant clinical experience and literally 160 hours of research interviews by this author, the coping "strategies" used most frequently by parents of technology assisted children are embodied in the statements often repeated: "You 'gotta' do what you 'gotta' do" and "Take it one day at a time," which seem to be largely internal or at the least compromises which had developed over time. For "when the sea was calm," said Shakespeare, "all boats alike showed mastership in floating" (White, 1974). That is, only in a storm are families obliged to "cope." When thinking of coping, what is generally implied is a fairly drastic change or problem that defies familiar ways of behaving, which very likely gives rise to uncomfortable affects like anxiety, guilt or grief, and which requires new ways of behaving or coping. Having "coped," people experience relief of discomfort and gradually adaptation develops out of subsequent situations. Hence, coping is adaptation in process and in relatively difficult circumstances (White, 1974).

When families of technology assisted infants and children who had been at home for a while were interviewed, what was probably being seen was "adaptation" to already existing, previously experienced circumstances and crises with which they had already "coped." Asking parents who had been at home for some years how they coped with various aspects of home care is tantamount to asking how they coped with buying groceries week in and week out. That is, much of what family members actually do to deal with the stress of home care over time is probably so second nature that it is no longer a consciously conceptualized process. Nonetheless, in order to work more effectively with families, it is important to have an overview of the process for those families experiencing long-term home care.

STAGES OF ADAPTATION

You learn what is "emergency" and what is not an emergency–I don't react as much anymore–I'm much more tolerant and patient than I used to be–If it's not life threatening then there's no reason to get bent out of shape.

There are stages which families of technology assisted infants and children seem to go through to achieve some semblance of normalcy. The first month at home seems to burn especially bright in the minds of many parents who repeatedly reiterate that "the first month of home care does not count because it is so awful." One father described it as being "like a cat on a hot tin roof, only it's a whole family of cats on a very hot tin roof." No matter how good the educational and training experience at the hospital to prepare families for home care, the first month is barely describable by most because it was so anxiety ridden.

The next five months also seem to be critical. The same father cited above described this period of time: "like being cats on a very warm roof which is basically tolerable but it could heat up at any given moment. You can live with it but it's not comfortable." Parents are clear that "if you can survive the first six months you can survive anything, including war and pestilence." They have indicated that it clearly took four to six months to be able to comfortably leave the house, resume normal sexual relationships with spouses and to generally resume other family and work-related activities without major anxiety. When asked what helps, parents attribute the decrease in anxiety to being successful in getting through the first major medical crisis or emergency with the child. Perhaps when parents were successful in being able to handle an emergency, to see that they could handle thinking and acting under extreme pressure, an additional layer of confidence was built. Some parents also attribute the decrease in anxiety to achieving consistency of coverage by nursing staff they felt they could trust with the child. However, it is also after the initial few months of home care that parents began to experience authority and control issues with the nurses. It appears that as parents gain in overall confidence, they begin to become more critical of the care the nurses are providing. They begin to rely less on the judgments of the nurses and to trust more in their own ability to determine the needs and care of the child. It is of interest that many families lose many of their "original" nurses at around the six month time either because the families ask nurses to leave or nurses choose to leave on their own.

Parents who do not start going out of the house in a fairly regular way within the first six months tend to become increasingly socially isolated. These parents may attribute their isolation to inconsistency of nursing and not having nurses who they felt they could trust, but also report that as home care progresses they simply do not have enough time, energy or resources for other activities.

After the first six months, the next 12 to 18 months of home care seem to be a time of relative calm, provided the staffing of nurses in the home are settled into a consistent pattern, supplies and equipment are on a schedule and the child is relatively stable in health. Although this time is characterized by increasing difficulties with nurses, parents experience more relative ease and everything seems to run a fairly normal course as defined by the situation.

The next critical time in the adaptation process to home care seems to be around the two-year point. At that time, many families seem to go through a crisis experience which is generally shown in two ways: increased marital discord; and increased conflict with nurses including the potential for the explosive firing of nurses and nursing agencies. From observing this consistent pattern and from talking with parents, it seems as though what is really going on is the realization that home care is going to be a long-term experience or at least that it was not going to go away for awhile. This realization is hard for families because there is the feeling that this knowledge had been dealt with or at least should have been dealt with before the child came home.

It is not clear why this relatively predictable yet sudden upheaval would occur two years into home care. Nonetheless, by applying developmental theory, this crisis time after a period of relative calm looks very much like the adolescent's struggle away from dependence on the family toward autonomy and independence in society. The family in home care seems to struggle away from dependence on the health care system toward autonomy and independence as a family unit. The conflictual nature of this struggle for independence from the "system" seems to be fueled by the competence parents gain in the two years of caring for their child. However, unlike the competence of the adolescent which does lead to independence from the family unit, the families' competence in home care does not lead to independence from the health care system. Parents seem to rail against the realization of this long-term dependence by attacking the most available and logical targets: each other and the nurses.

This crisis in home care does not go on ad infinitum because no one has the energy. It is at this point that it is possible to discern two basic forms of resolution at which families might arrive. One outcome was a sense of hopelessness and helplessness, seen in some families. However, for the most part, resolving the crisis seems to result in the family's reorganization toward the goals of "getting on with life" and moving forward with the family not so defined by the need to deal with the child's condition. There is a re-structuring of roles and responsibilities in the care of the child and a more conscious effort to "do" normal activities both with and without the child. More importantly, there is an acceptance that while some aspects of family life are going to be forever changed, the family doesn't have to be forever consumed. The resulting approaches to home care are epitomized by "you 'gotta' do what you 'gotta' do," and "take it one day at a time," which are clear indicators of this restructuring. It is after this crisis, for example, that mothers in particular tend to relinquish some of their "supervisory" responsibilities and rely more heavily on one home care nurse as the "charge nurse." There is a more general backing away from the nurses and although there continue to be some problems, having a designated line of authority seems to free up parents to be able to be "parents."

Based on this developmental process in home care, it seems logical that parents found dealing with the nurses in the home, the financial situation and the health of the child as the greatest sources of stress because they are likely to cause anxiety. From the parents' perspective, they are also the most insecure aspects of home care and illuminate most clearly the dependence on the health care system.

OCCUPATIONAL STRESS

> The care of (child) feels like it's more important than I am. So the result is a protective wall kind of thing so there are times of getting close which you know can only go so far–you'll be too emotionally involved and angry when the reality comes back that she (wife) will have to go and take care of (child).

It is not difficult to understand why having others in the home up to 18 hours a day would be stressful and affect family functioning. However, in thinking about why the difficulties with nurses would remain such a persistent problem, it seems that the lack of role definition and the lack of clearly delineated lines of authority are significant sources of problems. In pursuing this idea further, concepts such as role ambiguity, role conflict and role strain, as found in the occupational stress literature, seem to be particularly relevant to the problems parents experience with nurses in the home.

Kahn and his colleagues (1964) focused on the existence of occupational stress resulting from conflicting, incompatible or unclear expectations in the work environment. They found that "role conflict" occurred when the expected behaviors of employees were inconsistent with demands. The inconsistency resulted most often when a single employee had multiple supervisors and was put in the position of being in the middle of conflicting demands from different sources. When the employee was expected to be doing tasks which were in conflict or when there was the demand to do multiple tasks at the same time, the individual would experience conflict and stress.

On the other hand, "role ambiguity" derives from a lack of necessary information regarding position within the organization and a lack of information regarding the actual role. For Pearlin (1983), events can create stress because they adversely alter or intensify the more enduring aspects of key social roles. It is the altered social roles which, in turn, produce stress. Most roles exist within such institutions as family, occupation, economy and education. Since people are typically socialized to invest themselves rather heavily in these roles, any problems are potent sources of stress and cannot be ignored.

Using Kahn's description of role conflict and ambiguity and Pearlin's concepts of altered social roles, it becomes possible to understand why there seemed to be such consistent stress between parents and skilled care providers in the home. The social roles which Pearlin identifies as of most critical importance are those of provider and family member. It is impossible for these roles to be unaffected by the home care situation and it seems that at the heart of the "stress with nurses" is the lack of clarity in "job description." When parents and nurses are both doing nursing as well as parenting tasks, it seems only logical that there will be role strain. Nurses are paid care providers who work eight hour shifts, while parents must pay out-of-pocket for the opportunity to perform the same tasks as the nurses. Parents are ultimately responsible for care 24 hours a day, seven days a week, so when a nurse fails to come to work, very often the parents are the "back up." While parents of "normal" children also must take responsibility for their children on a full time basis and not get paid for "parenting," there is not the glaring inequity in responsibility and reward as exists between nurses and parents in home care of the technology assisted child. The nurse goes home at the end of the shift; for the parent, the work is in the home and there is little relief. Similarly, in the role as "breadwinner," parents often feel inadequate to be able to meet the financial demands of home care and stress at work often impedes parents' ability to meet the emotional demands of the home care situation.

The role captivity inherent in home care is obvious both in and out of the home as the freedom to move, change jobs or "just be a parent" are not true options. Re-structuring of family relationships is necessary with the influx of multiple care providers, decreased financial status and the morass of information with which parents must deal on a daily basis. Parents must take on a large number of roles, such as financial planner, personnel manager, and respiratory, physical and occupational therapists, such that the lines of demarcation between "parenting" and "managing care" are often non-existent.

In the past, the home has been viewed as a place of employment for the home care nurse and not conceptually considered to be a place of "employment" for the parents. If the vocabulary, however, is shifted from "place of employment" to "work place" then it becomes easier to understand why, for example, there was conflict over the manner in which care was provided and who was in control of decision making about the child. In light of "role conflict" and "role ambiguity" one can see why "staff meetings," memos, organized orientation and training and a communication notebook might work well to negotiate, structure and define roles as well as communication between parents and nurses.

Concepts related to occupational stress also help to explain why, for example, parents talk about not having any vacation or time off from the care of the child and feel they should be paid for covering shifts which a nurse missed. It explains why parents have arrived at the understanding that it is better not to be friends with the nurses but rather to maintain an "employer/employee" relationship. This would also explain why parents and especially mothers define their lives in terms of nursing shifts and schedules of treatments. While there is certainly a practical side to this method of operating, the view of parenting the medically fragile child as "occupation" begins to expose some of the seemingly impersonal behaviors of parents, e.g., communicating through notebooks, the posting rules and regulations, and anger for having to cover nursing shifts, for what they might in reality be: reactions to role conflict, role ambiguity, role strain and role captivity at "work."

These role related concepts do not only apply to parents and nurses. Siblings are thoroughly unsure of where they fit into the picture with their parents and the nurses, if at all. They feel isolated from the technology assisted child and are unclear on what role they have in the life of their brother or sister. The technology assisted children also have to learn to adjust to the role of long-term dependence, at a developmental time when independence is the objective. Thus, even the children in the families where there is a technology assisted child experience role strain and personal stress in trying to establish their own roles within the family. The myriad of role changes and potential areas of stress and strain inherent in having nurses in the home gives credence to the consideration of the theories related to occupational stress.

Family members do learn to cope with the various crises and anxieties of the early months of home care and achieve a level of acceptance of the situation. This acceptance or adaptation to home care provides families with the internal protection they needed to deal with the extraordinary circumstances of pediatric home care so that the extraordinary will become ordinary. Families learn to live with and tolerate a higher level of anxiety after the first six months which enables them to normalize and redefine their lives to accommodate a higher level of stress than existed prior to home care. While specific coping strategies used by family members to reach this point have not been adequately studied, the fact that most families do cope reasonably well and do accommodate over time is an important recognition.

CONCLUSION

We've walked through hell together and have survived together. It's made us stronger as a couple, while at the same time put a lot of cracks in the marriage also. We've survived some severe blows.

Overall, despite the difficulties, parents definitely feel the benefits of home care outweigh the problems and limitations. They also feel that there were benefits for the other children in the family but acknowledge the negative impact on siblings. Siblings also are articulate about their mixed feelings about home care. While they tend to be careful not to blame the technology assisted child, they feel left out of the family and less important to their parents than the technology assisted child. Despite this, they also feel they benefit by becoming more tolerant of other people, more knowledgeable about medical information and more responsible than if they had not had the experience of home care. So while it is easy to see many of the negatives of home care, the family members' perceptions of the positive changes in family relationships and the overall benefits of home care add an important dimension to working with these families.

At a micro level, there are numerous concrete issues inherent in helping families with an infant or child dependent on life support technology, including: learning the technical skills; educational planning; social and familial supports; emergency planning and so forth. But at a macro or a larger systems level, it is important to enable parents to have the information and the skills they need to maintain family functioning while trying to make "ordinary" an extraordinary circumstance. This means enabling parents to remain as a family while becoming managers of their child and family. This includes the need for information and the skills necessary to deal "occupationally" with the other systems which enter their lives; support for the ongoing "process" of home care as family members learn to adapt; and, support for the "negative" side of home care as well as the positive. While developmentally, "home" is the best place for any infant or child, it is not simply a "there's no place like home" experience for the family. We need to acknowledge that and help parents to weigh the costs and the benefits not just for the child with special needs, but for all the family members.

Accepted for Publication: 05/14/96

REFERENCES

Andrews, G., Tennant, C., Hewson, D., and Vaillant, G.: Life event stress, social support, coping styles and risk of psychological impairment. Journal of Nervous and Mental Disease 166: 307-316, 1978.

Barbarin, O.A., Hughes, D., and Chesler, M.A.: Stress, coping, and marital functioning among parents of children with cancer. Journal of Marriage and the Family 47(2): 473-80, 1985.

Bone, R.C.: Long term ventilator care: A Chicago problem and a national problem. Chest 93(3): 536-539, 1987.

Brimblecombe, F.S.W.: The needs of parents of young handicapped children living at home. In Stress and Disability in Childhood: The Long Term Problems, eds. N.R. Butler and D.D. Corner, pp. 78-86. Bristol: Wright, 1984.

Children's Home Health Network of Illinois (CHHNI): Project Summary for Year 1984. Agency document of DSCC, Chicago, IL, 1984.

Children's Home Health Network of Illinois (CHHNI): Project Final Report. Model of Discharge and Home Care Planning. Agency document of DSCC, 1987.

Coffman, S.P.: Parents' perceptions of needs for themselves and their children in a cerebral palsy clinic. Issues in Comprehensive Pediatric Nursing 6: 67-77, 1983.

Figley, C.: Catastrophes: An overview of family reactions. In Stress and the Family: Volume II: Coping with Catastrophe, eds. H. McCubbin and C. Figley, pp. 3-20. New York: Brunner/Mazel, 1983.

Gallagher, J.J., Beckman, P., and Cross, A.H.: Families of handicapped children: Sources of stress and its amelioration. Exceptional Children 50(1): 10-19, 1983.

Goldberg, A., Faure, E., and Vaughn, C.: Home care for life supported persons: An approach to program development. Journal of Pediatrics 104: 785-795, 1984.

Hochstadt, N. and Yost, D., (Eds.): The Medically Complex Child: The Transition to Home. New York: Harwood, 1991.

Horner, M.M., Rawlins, P., and Giles, K.: How parents of children with chronic conditions perceive their own needs. Maternal and Child Nursing 12(1): 40-43, 1987.

Kahn, R.L., Wolfe, D.M., Quinn, R.P., and Snoek, J.D.: Organizational Stress: Studies in Role Conflict and Ambiguity. New York: John Wiley and Sons, Inc., 1964.

Kazak, A.E.: Families with physically handicapped children: Social ecology and family systems. Family Process 25(2): 265-281, 1986.

McCubbin, H.I., Larson, A., and Olson, D.H.: Family crisis oriented personal evaluation scales. In Family Inventories, revised edition. MN: University of Minnesota, Family Social Science, 290 McNeal Ave., St. Paul, Minnesota, 1981.

McCubbin, H.I. and Figley, C.: Bridging normative and catastrophic family stress. In Stress and the Family: Volume I: Coping with Normative Transitions, eds. H.I. McCubbin and C.R. Figley, pp. 218-228. New York: Brunner/Mazel, 1983.

McCubbin, H.I. and Patterson, J.M.: Family transitions: Adaptation to stress. In Stress and the Family, Volume I: Coping with Normative Transitions, eds. H.I. McCubbin and C.R. Figley. New York: Brunner/Mazel, 1983.

McCubbin, M.: Nursing assessment of parental coping with cystic fibrosis. Western Journal of Nursing Research 6(4): 407-418, 1984.

Menaghan, E.G.: Individual coping efforts: Moderators of the relationship between life stress and mental health outcomes. Psychological Stress: Trends in Theory and Research, ed. Howard B. Kaplan, pp. 105-155. New York: Academic Press, 1983.

Morris, L.W. and Engle, W.B.: Assessing various coping strategies and their effects on test performance. Journal of Clinical Psychology 37: 165-171, 1981.

Office of Technology Assessment (OTA) Report: Technology Dependent Children: Hospital vs Home care. Technical Memorandum. U.S. Congress, Washington, D.C. #OTA-TM-H-38, 1987.

Pearlin, L.I.: Role strain and personal stress. Psychosocial Stress: Trends in Theory and Research, ed. H.B. Kaplan. New York: Academic Press, 1983.

Pearlin, L.I. and Schooler, C.: The structure of coping. Journal of Health and Social Behavior 22: 337-356, 1978.

Rehabilitation Institute of Chicago, National Foundation-March of Dimes, Care for Life, and Rehabilitation Gazette. What ever happened to the polio patient? Proceedings of the international symposium. Chicago, Illinois, Oct 14-16, 1981.

Report of the Brook Lodge invitational symposium on the ventilator dependent child. Augusta, Michigan. October 16-18, 1983. Upjohn Health Care Services, 2605 E. Kilgore Road, Kalamazoo, MI 49002, 1983.

Stein, R.E.K. and Jessop, D.: Evaluation of a home care unit as an ambulatory ICU. Final report, grant #: MC-R360402 of the Maternal and Child Health and Crippled Children's grants program. Rockville, MD 20857, 1984.

Stuifbergen, A.K.: The impact of chronic illness on families. Family and Community Health 9(4): 43-51, 1987.

Taylor, S.C.: The effect of chronic illnesses upon well siblings. Maternal and Child Nursing Journal 9: 109-116, 1980.

Turner, R.J.: Direct, indirect, and moderating effects of social support on psychological distress and associated conditions. In Psychological Stress: Trends in Theory and Research, ed. H.B. Kaplan, pp. 105-155. New York: Academic Press, 1983.

USDHHS. Report of the Surgeon General's Workshop on Children with Handicaps and Their Families. DHHS Pub #PHS-83-50194 Washington, DC: U.S. Govt Printing Office, 1982.

USDHHS. Infantile apnea and home monitoring. Report of a Consensus Development Conference, September 29, 30, and October 1, 1986. Vol. 6(6). NIH Publication #87-2905, Bethesda, Maryland, 1987.

White, R.W.: Strategies of adaptation: An attempt at systematic description. In Coping and Adaptation, eds. G. Coelho, D. Hamburg, and J. Adams, pp. 47-68. New York: Basic Books, Inc., 1974.

The Profile of HIV Infection in Women:
A Challenge to the Profession

Debra A. Katz, MSW, LCSW

SUMMARY. Human Immunodeficiency Virus (HIV) has become a leading cause of morbidity and mortality among women and children in the United States. As advances are made in the area of diagnosis and treatment of HIV infection, strategies must be developed to support the psychosocial needs of women with HIV disease. The diagnosis of HIV infection in women and their children presents a unique array of complicated social, emotional and medical consequences. Care must be provided in a holistic manner with special emphasis on the needs of women within a systemic context. *[Article copies available for a fee from The Haworth Document Delivery Service: 1-800-342-9678. E-mail address: getinfo@haworth.com]*

HIV infection has become an epidemic of immense proportions, affecting people of every race, culture and economic level. The complex social, ethical, psychological and physical problems confronting people with HIV infection set it apart from any other disease.

The epidemiology of this disease is changing as the percentage of women with HIV infection increases steadily. Women are presently the fastest growing group of people with AIDS, with minority women and their children being disproportionately affected (Redman, 1990). AIDS is increasing four times as fast among women than men with more women presently being infected through heterosexual sex than drug use (Ward,

---

Debra A. Katz is AIDS Program Coordinator in the City of Stamford, CT.

[Haworth co-indexing entry note]: "The Profile of HIV Infection in Women: A Challenge to the Profession." Katz, Debra A. Co-published simultaneously in *Social Work in Health Care* (The Haworth Press, Inc.) Vol. 24, No. 3/4, 1997, pp. 127-134; and: *Fundamentals of Perinatal Social Work: A Guide for Clinical Practice with Women, Infants, and Families* (ed: Regina Furlong Lind, and Debra Honig Bachman) The Haworth Press, Inc., 1997, pp. 127-134. Single or multiple copies of this article are available for a fee from The Haworth Document Delivery Service [1-800-342-9678, 9:00 a.m. - 5:00 p.m. (EST). E-mail address: getinfo@haworth.com].

1993). In nine cities nationwide, AIDS is the leading cause of death for women 25-44 (Selik, Chu, Buehler, 1993).

AIDS is a serious crises for women; they are bearing the impact of this epidemic whether they are family, lovers or friends of persons with HIV, as women with AIDS or HIV, as professional caregivers or as HIV educators and advocates (Watstein and Laurich, 1991). The public perception of AIDS as a disease affecting gay males or injection drug users has significantly impacted on women's lack of adequate HIV education and the denial of their susceptibility to HIV infection. Many women remain unaware of their personal risk of contracting and spreading HIV infection. The majority of women with AIDS are single, economically disadvantaged and minority with multiproblem services needs (Greene and Springer, 1989). AIDS disproportionately affects women with the fewest resources and historically the most discriminated against in our society.

HIV INFECTION IN WOMEN

Women must identify the behaviors that put them at risk for HIV and not whether they are part of a particular high risk group. The primary behaviors that put women at risk for HIV infection are the sharing of needles or anal, vaginal or oral sex without a latex barrier condom (Ybarra, 1991).

A woman is at least ten times more susceptible to contracting HIV during intercourse than a man. This increased vulnerability is the result of the higher concentration of HIV in semen compared to vaginal fluid and the likely possibility that the vagina or labia is more prone to tiny cuts, tears or sores giving infected semen a route to enter the body (Patlak, 1993).

A woman's repeated unprotected sexual contact with one infected partner will increase her chances of becoming infected, but at the same time the more sexual partners a woman has the more likely it is that she can be exposed to HIV (Richardson, 1988).

Women have unique concerns with respect to HIV diagnosis and treatment. The diagnosis of HIV/AIDS in women usually occurs much later in the course of their illness than in men (Paolillo, 1992). Women seek treatment later because their health is often on the bottom of their list of priorities, which is further exacerbated by lack of insurance, lack of primary care providers and the absence of child care. A study done in New York City showed that more women are admitted to the hospital with their first AIDS related illness through the emergency room than men and far fewer women have private health insurance.

A study done at the University of Massachusetts Medical School and Cornell Medical Center found that most women seek medical attention a year after the diagnosis of HIV, and present at an advanced stage of their HIV infection. In addition, most women are not tested until a child or partner develops symptoms (Caschetta, 1992).

Women are often underdiagnosed for HIV/AIDS because of a failure by medical providers to look at HIV as a possible cause for medical complaints. Since men and their health care providers are more aware of the possibility of men contracting HIV, their diagnosis may occur at an earlier stage (Ybarra, 1991). Women's symptoms are often viewed differently than men's. A woman's reporting of weight loss, headaches and fatigue are more likely to be diagnosed as stress than if a man reported these symptoms.

In this country the majority of women are seen for health complaints in public health clinics, gynecologist offices or the emergency room. This kind of health care often leads to limited laboratory tests and diagnostic procedures which may result in the absence of adequate and ongoing medical data. The focus of a woman's care is usually related to a reproductive condition or her children's health care (Paolillo, 1992). The lack of attention to health care needs of women is not new. Gynecology has long been segregated from general medicine. Gynecologic concerns and their life threatening potential are often deemphasized and neglected (Marte and Allen, 1991). The common catch-22 for women is that OB/GYN specialists often are not HIV knowledgeable and infectious disease specialists are often not experienced in gynecological procedures and conditions. Further, if a woman is not considered by a health care provider to be a drug user or prostitute, HIV infection is often not even considered as a cause for the woman's presenting symptomatology.

In addition to all the HIV related illnesses that women have in common with men, women also have unique gynecologic manifestations of HIV diseases. These include: vaginal candidiasis, human papillomavirus and pelvic inflammatory disease.

Vaginal candidiasis (yeast infections) is the most common treatable gynecologic disorder for all women. However, for HIV infected women it is recurrent, difficult to treat and often the most frequent early sign of HIV disease in women. Human Papillomavirus Virus is the causative agent for genital warts as well as for cervical cancer. Treatment of genital warts for HIV infected women requires a long frustrating course of treatment yet the recurrence of the warts after this treatment is much more common for HIV infected women than for those uninfected. Cervical dysplasia, the precursor to cervical cancer, occurs at an unusually high rate in HIV infected women. Many of these women are not aware of this condition in time to get the necessary treatment to prevent cervical cancer, which is potentially fatal. Abnormal pap smears in HIV infected women is five to ten times the expected rate. Many providers feel HIV infected women should have pap smears every six months. Successful treatment of syphilis and herpes in HIV infected persons is difficult and often unsuccessful. These conditions will recur and more aggressive treatment will become necessary to prevent serious complications (Marte and Allen, 1991). Pelvic Inflammatory Disease is usually more severe and more common for women with HIV. Immediate hospitalization is recommended. Early detection and management of HIV infection, specifically gynecological conditions, in women is critical to improve their survival (Paolillo, 1992). Unusual or severe gynecological conditions which are unresponsive to treatment should alert practitioners that HIV infection should be considered.

Progression of HIV disease in women still remains fairly unexplored and only recently are studies being done to compare the natural history of HIV in men and women. One cannot assume that what we have learned for men is applicable to women. Act Up in New York reported that women are under-represented in clinical trials of experimental HIV/AIDS drugs in the United States. Of all national trials as of January 16, 1992, only 1,151 women had participated in drug trials for HIV/AIDS. This represents 7.8% of all drug trial slots. If a drug trial is to detect clinically significant gender differences in toxicities and response to therapy, the representative sample size for women must be greater than 15% (Caschetta, 1992). Women have often been excluded or discouraged from research studies. Reasons cited include: not enough women with AIDS to make it significantly accurate, researchers want to study uniform populations such as men, or the potential harm to a woman's reproductive capacity or a fetus during pregnancy. Clinical trials are often insensitive to women's special needs for childcare or transportation. Recruitment of HIV infected women to drug trials is also limited since most referrals are through private medical care and most HIV infected women use public hospitals or clinics. Little effort is made to inform seropositive women of available clinical trials. HIV infected women with infected children must often negotiate four different providers in four locations: her routine provider, her clinical trial site, her child's routine provider and her child's clinical site. Even a woman with extraordinary resources would find this task difficult. For the average HIV infected woman who must worry about food, clothing and shelter, this task is nearly impossible. Efforts to increase access to HIV clinical trials for women will only be successful if they are integrated into the same site as medical care for both women and children (Paolillo 1992). New aggressive combination treatments appear to have the ability to significantly improve the quality and quantity of one's life with HIV, thus making access to care even more vital.

PERINATAL COUNSELING

HIV counseling and testing during prenatal care can assist in identifying HIV infection in pregnant women. Knowledge of a pregnant woman's HIV status can provide early diagnosis and treatment for mother and child, help a woman make informed reproductive choices, reduce the risk of perinatal transition and provide for referral to vital services.

CDC (Center of Disease Control) has published guidelines recommending routine regularly offered HIV counseling and voluntary HIV testing on all pregnant women. HIV counseling should become a routine part of prenatal care, which would begin to remove the stigma associated with HIV testing. Pregnant women who receive quality and empathic HIV counseling are able to make an informed decision regarding HIV testing. Experience has demonstrated that over 95% of pregnant women, if offered routine HIV counseling and voluntary HIV testing, will choose to take the test.

Concerns arise when considering the option of mandatory prenatal HIV testing. Mandatory testing could result in fear and distrust of providers, non-compliance with prenatal care or lack of commitment to HIV treatment recommendations.

The discussion of HIV testing for newborns and pregnant women has accelerated since the release in June, 1994 of the results of the 076 clinical trials. This study showed that selected pregnant women who were given ZDV (AZT) during pregnancy, during labor and delivery and to the newborn after birth demonstrated a reduction in the risk of perinatal transmission of HIV to their newborns by approximately two-thirds: 8.3% of those born to mothers who received ZDV were infected compared to 25.5% of infants born to mothers in the control group who did not receive ZDV (Conner, Sperling, Gelber et al., 1994).

Pregnant women with HIV infection must be able to obtain information on both the benefits and potential risks of receiving ZDV therapy. A collaborative approach by the medical team and counselor is needed to help these women reach a decision that will help both their newborn and themselves.

PSYCHOSOCIAL ISSUES

The unique psychosocial needs of women can be divided into four categories: individual, relationship, mothering and pregnancy.

An HIV positive woman may grieve for her loss of health, body image, sexuality, femininity and childbearing potential. She may feel guilty for past behaviors and view the illness as a punishment. Seropositive women often feel shame related to sexuality and will withdraw from relationships for fear of being rejected and abandoned (Ybarra, 1991). Unique to women is the female social role of mothering. When a woman with HIV infection becomes ill, her role as caretaker for her children and other family members is affected and therefore severely disrupts the functioning of the family (Shaw, 1987).

Many women do not learn of their own HIV infection until their child is diagnosed. A mother's shock may soon lead to denial. This denial can result in medical neglect of their child and themselves. This state of denial can also impact on a woman's decision to get pregnant since the threat of an infected infant is not acknowledged. For many of these women, childbearing is a cultural expectation and a sign of their worth. HIV infected women who choose to forego childbearing will experience a profound sense of loss and will grieve over the child they never had (Ybarra, 1991).

Self blame for women with HIV can become intolerable if children are involved. If the children are healthy, the mother may also feel grief stricken at the thought of having to leave them behind. If the child is infected, the mother will often feel overwhelming guilt and blame. Many HIV infected mothers may become too sick to care for their own children and must plan for their welfare and future. Some mothers may even have to watch their children die as they wait for their own death (Ybarra, 1991).

COUNSELING IMPLICATIONS

In counseling women with HIV infection, mental health providers must be aware of their own assumptions and prejudices. The majority of these women are poor and from minority communities; therefore, cultural sensitivity is vital. HIV resources and services must address ethnic concerns and attitudes. Providers must be comfortable with issues of sexuality, substance abuse and death.

Helping women to cope with the diagnosis of HIV requires acceptance and listening as these women deal with their feelings of anger, shame, guilt, blame and depression. For HIV infected women with few resources and overwhelming environmental stresses, psychological insight may be limited. Support and active case management will assist HIV infected women in meeting their medical and psychosocial needs. It is crucial to stress hope by helping HIV infected women to maintain control of their lives as well as good health practices. Emotional support is needed to help these women with their feelings of worthlessness, fear of abandonment, isolation and helplessness. Promoting a woman's self esteem and dignity will result in the validation of her own self worth and self empowerment. Grief work must be interwoven throughout the counseling process. HIV infected women must be assisted in self forgiveness and in recognizing their losses. Profound despair must be redirected so that these women can reinvest their energy in the challenges ahead. Counselors must carefully assess the suicide potential of their clients and take necessary treatment steps as needed.

HIV infection will place great strains on a woman's relationships. Issues of safer sex, disclosing HIV status and partner notification must be discussed at length.

Women with HIV infection must make an informed decision about their reproductive options. They have a right to all information about HIV disease and pregnancy so they can make this very personal decision. This counseling process must be both individualized to match each person's coping mechanisms and ongoing since HIV information changes rapidly. After providing information, answering questions and emphasizing that much about HIV and pregnancy is still not known, a woman is still left with a very difficult and personal decision.

For women who have HIV infected children, counseling must focus on issues of guilt and self blame. Women must be assisted in forgiving themselves before they die. Women must be empowered to help make arrangements for their HIV infected or healthy children. Placement arrangements with relatives, or foster care must be explored. Mothers who are struggling with their own grief and guilt may find it hard to talk to their children about HIV and dying. Honesty is difficult but essential and if children are old enough to ask questions, they must be answered.

Professionals must have a forum to express and explore their own feelings in working with persons with HIV infection. With gaps in available services, providers can feel helpless in meeting the needs of their clients. As providers, our own personal conflicts can arise in regard to the client's behaviors that led to their infection or a mother's perinatal transmission to her children. Working with young clients who eventually will suffer and die will make us feel vulnerable. As social work professionals, our challenge is to be compassionate providers and leaders in advocating for the needs of those with HIV infection.

Accepted for Publication: 05/15/96

REFERENCES

Bermon, N, MD. (1993). Family and Reproductive Issues. *AIDS Clinical Care*, 5(6), 45-47.

Caschetta, M. (1992). A Review of Reports on Women and HIV. *Treatment Issues*, 6(10), 2-8.

Conner, E., Sperling, R., Gelber, R. et al. (1994). Reduction of maternal-infant transmission of human immunodeficiency virus type with zidovudine treatment. *New England Journal Medicine*, 331:1173-1180.

Greene, E., Springer, E. (1989). Women and AIDS: Who Takes Care of the Women? *Womens Action Alliance Inc.*

Marte, C., MD, Allen, M., MD. (1991). HIV Related Gynecological Conditions: Overlooked Complications. *Focus A Guide to AIDS Research and Counseling*, 7(1), 1-4.

Paolillo, L., Ph.D. (1992). Women and AIDS. *Provincetown Positive*, 13:1-18.

Patlak, M. (1993). AIDS Is a Women's Issue. *New Woman*, 67-70.

Pinsky, L., Douglas, P. (1992). *The Essential HIV Treatment Fact Book*. New York: Simon & Schuster.

Quackenbush, M., Sargent, P. (1990). *Teaching AIDS*. California: ETR Associates.

Redman, J., MSW, MPH. (1990). Women and AIDS: What We Need to Know. *Planned Parenthood Resource Material*.

Richardson, D. (1988). *Women and AIDS*. New York: Methuen Inc.

Selik, R., MD, Chu, S., Ph.D., Buehler, J., MD. (1993). HIV Infection as Leading Cause of Death Among Young Adults in U.S. Cities and States. *JAMA*, 269(23), 2991-2994.

Shaw, N., Ph.D. (1987). AIDS: Special Concerns for Women (pp. 123-125). *Working with AIDS: A Resource Guide for Mental Health Professionals*. University of California, San Francisco. pp. 123-125.

Wara, D., MD. (1993). Pediatric AIDS: Perinatal Transmission and Early Diagnosis. *AIDS Clinical Care*, 5(3), 21.

Ward, J., MD. (1993). *Centers for Disease Control and Prevention Report*.

Watstein, S., Laurich, R. (1991). *AIDS and Women*. Arizona: The Oryx Press.

Weedy, C., MSW. (1993). Psychosocial Issues in Pediatric AIDS. *NCMJ*, 54(1), 18-23.

Ybarra, Sharon. (1991). Women and AIDS: Implications for Counseling. *Journal of Counseling and Development*, 69:285-287.

Social Policy Considerations in Perinatal Social Work

Carol K. Mahan, MSW

SUMMARY. Infant mortality has been a major problem in the United States for many years. Despite recent improvements, it continues to be a major social and economic problem. This is particularly true in non-white populations, where the infant mortality rate is significantly higher. This article discusses some of the reasons for the continued high rate of infant mortality, with particular attention to barriers which, if removed, might improve the health of newborn infants. How social workers can use this information in advocacy efforts is then explored in an effort to involve social workers more directly in this pressing national problem. *[Article copies available for a fee from The Haworth Document Delivery Service: 1-800-342-9678. E-mail address: getinfo@haworth.com]*

The debate about health care reform over the past few years has been both frustrating and heartening. Frustrating because it produced few tangible results, but heartening in that, finally, this issue is getting some broader, national attention. Aspects of the debate, particularly those which focused on access to care and disease prevention, undoubtedly raised awareness in sectors of our society which previously ignored these important considerations. Although the debate covered the gamut of health care

Carol K. Mahan is affiliated with West Park Hospital, 707 Sheridan Avenue, Cody, WY 82414.

This paper is adapted from "Infant Mortality: Implications for Social Work and Social Policy," NAPSW FORUM, Spring, 1990.

[Haworth co-indexing entry note]: "Social Policy Considerations in Perinatal Social Work." Mahan, Carol K. Co-published simultaneously in *Social Work in Health Care* (The Haworth Press, Inc.) Vol. 24, No. 3/4, 1997, pp. 135-140; and: *Fundamentals of Perinatal Social Work: A Guide for Clinical Practice with Women, Infants, and Families* (ed: Regina Furlong Lind, and Debra Honig Bachman) The Haworth Press, Inc., 1997, pp. 135-140. Single or multiple copies of this article are available for a fee from The Haworth Document Delivery Service [1-800-342-9678, 9:00 a.m. - 5:00 p.m. (EST). E-mail address: getinfo@haworth.com].

concerns, there was welcome attention to the problems of infant mortality and morbidity, childhood illnesses and other maternal-child health concerns. While there have been continuing improvements in overall infant mortality over the past several years (from 10.6/1000 births in 1985 to 7.9/1000 in 1994), the improvements are not reflected proportionately among population groups. In 1992, black infants were 2.4 times more likely to die than white infants, with mortality rates of 16.5 and 6.9 respectively, per 1000 live births (Billings, 1995; Casey, 1994). Further, improvements in infant mortality more than likely reflect technological improvements in the treatment of premature and otherwise ill newborns, rather than prevention of prematurity and babies with other conditions requiring neonatal intensive care. Thus, a discussion of infant mortality is useful and illustrative when examining broad perinatal health care issues, and subsequently, relevant roles for social workers in the amelioration of such social policy stagnation.

When examining the U.S. infant mortality rate it is tempting to search for a single, obvious cause, rather than the multiple, often subtle causal factors which are involved. Undoubtedly, a major problem remains access to care. Barriers to access are partially financial, which is unfortunate and short sighted, since a few hundred dollars spent per pregnancy for prenatal care can avoid the prolonged hospitalization of a low birth-weight baby, at an average of $150,000/stay. The cost-benefit ratio of prenatal care would seem quite clear (Healthy, 1989; Governing, 1988).

But in truth, the problems associated with access are complex, and go beyond finances. The mere presence or absence of prenatal clinics is an insufficient measure of the availability of services to poor pregnant women. As Florida Governor Lawton Chiles stated while serving in the U.S. Senate, "Access can be denied in a number of ways: through cultural inhibitions, through inconvenience, through lack of money, or through lack of knowledge" (Raspberry, 1989).

In fact, if the physical presence of health care clinics was the only access issue, cities with neighborhood clinics, such as Detroit and Washington, D.C., would not continue to suffer infant mortality rates of nearly 20 infants per 1000 live births. In reality, access to care involves many facets, including qualification for Medicaid or other assistance programs. Few states offer comprehensive "one stop" services, in which clients can learn about, complete applications and qualify for relevant programs. Transportation to and from scheduled appointments, and child care for other children during health care appointments are barriers which, for many patients, are no less formidable than the actual lack of health related programs.

Although access is an important barrier, it is one of several intertwined issues which must be considered. Perinatal substance abuse is an increasing factor in infant mortality and morbidity, and is linked to an access issue of another type–access to substance abuse treatment programs. Many programs exclude pregnant women from participation, and few programs exist specifically for this population. Further, recent federal budgets, though they have included significant funding increases for drug related problems, have earmarked drug enforcement rather than drug treatment or drug awareness education. It is perhaps illustrative of the tendency in this country to fix, rather than prevent, the problem.

Education must also be considered. Educational initiatives are not always effective, or targeted at the populations most in need of learning, for example, about the efficacy of prenatal care. Unfortunately, too many educational programs, such as those promoting condom use in disease prevention, are drastically altered to gain acceptance among the more conservative segments of local communities.

There are many other issues which could illustrate the failure of social policy to keep pace with clearly identified societal need: adolescent pregnancy, child hunger, juvenile crime, single parent families and homelessness, to name a few. Hardly an exhaustive list, the above is meant to spur thinking about all that must be done to reduce infant mortality, morbidity and associated social problems, and to ensure that our nation's children will have a healthy start in life.

THE INVOLVEMENT OF SOCIAL WORKERS IN SOCIAL POLICY ISSUES

Concern with social issues is a value inherent in the social work profession. That concern has often been in the form of working with individuals and/or families to help make their existence a better one. Increasingly, social workers have individually and collectively worked to improve the system for a greater number of persons. Organizations such as NASW have a long history of sensitivity to and activism on behalf of the disadvantaged and the social policy issues which affect them. NASW and other such organizations have advocated for everything from access to health care to peace, justice and human rights issues.

The National Association of Perinatal Social Workers (NAPSW) is a much newer and smaller organization. Its roots in social policy issues are less deep, but are at the core of many issues facing our country and its children. NAPSW began primarily as an educational organization, but entered the social policy arena when "Baby Doe," a handicapped newborn whose parents chose not to treat, became a household name. With the organization's first letter to then President Reagan in 1983, the Social Action Committee was formed to address that and subsequent pressing social and ethical concerns. Because of their unique focus on perinatal health issues, NAPSW's efforts have been more narrowly defined than those of other groups (e.g., NASW or the Children's Defense Fund) and are largely limited to issues of pregnancy, childbirth and infancy. Within that arena, however, lie some powerful and often controversial issues, such as abortion, adoption and the treatment of newborns with birth defects.

Over the past decade, NAPSW has supported a variety of legislative efforts with emphasis on strengthening the family. The organization has uniformly opposed legislation which would withdraw support–financial, practical or emotional–from families. The preponderance of effort organizationally has been at the federal level, primarily on pending legislation. State and local issues, and cases before the courts have been targeted less often; however, some have been the subject of attention due to their ramifications for the broader system.

PRIORITIZING PERINATAL HEALTH

Although most persons would support the importance of a healthy start for our country's infants, it is elevating this issue to its rightful place of prominence that is the challenge for social workers. Japan, the country ranked lowest in infant mortality in the world, did so in 1951, by proclaiming their "Children's Charter." Among other points, it states that "All children shall be assured of healthy minds and bodies and shall be guaranteed freedom from want" and "All children shall be provided with adequate nourishment, housing, and clothing and shall be protected against disease and injury" (Japan, 1951). Their efforts have obviously been successful, as evidenced by their infant mortality ranking, and they can serve as a model country which has truly prioritized children's health, with all of the economic and educational support from the public and private sector that such an effort requires.

Although Japan leads the way, it would be unfair to imply that there are no successful programs within the U.S. Some areas and programs are doing well, or have made great strides in previously problematic areas. Our challenge is to learn from them, and to apply this wisdom elsewhere, with adaptations to meet the individual needs of particular communities and populations.

IMPLICATIONS FOR SOCIAL WORKERS

There are so many unmet needs, one can become overwhelmed with all that requires attention. However, no problems are unresolvable, and the efforts of one individual or program cannot be underestimated. Certainly, among health care providers in the perinatal field, social workers are in a unique position to understand the impact of social problems on health care issues. Appropriate roles for perinatal social workers may include any or all of the following:

- Spend time educating others, including the media, government officials, other health care professionals and the general public. Help them understand the extent to which social problems affect or become medical problems. But stop "preaching to the saved"–spend your time and energy on different groups than you might have in the past. Targeting private industry or service groups not directly associated with perinatal issues can produce greater results than you might expect.
- Join groups or committees which are actively trying to influence the system. Whether that system is a governmental entity or a private enterprise, you can join with others for a greater impact.
- Try the grass roots approach. Write letters or make calls to your elected representatives or others with influence in health care. Once you have done it enough to demystify the process, it is enjoyable. You might be surprised to learn the influence you can have as well as the level of interest on the part of elected officials.
- Work with consumers and consumer groups–they wield much more influence than they realize. For example, letters to politicians from parents of low birth weight babies (especially with pictures) can really make a difference. Many consumers, particularly those not associated with organizations, need encouragement to get started, but are glad to help. Local parent support organizations can be a great resource for you, and are often seen as less self serving than health care professionals.
- Support voter registration and candidate awareness in poor or medically underserved areas. Babies don't vote, but it helps to empower those who do and are most in need of assistance programs and expanded health care services.
- Work with organizations such as NAPSW, NASW and the Children's Defense Fund, and collaborate with other organizations sharing similar priorities.

It is important not to underestimate the influence that one person can have. Whether you influence one individual client or pending legislation that ultimately affects millions, take heart in knowing that your efforts have helped make life better for at least one potential leader of tomorrow.

Accepted for Publication: 05/14/96

REFERENCES

Billings Gazette. (1995). US Infant Mortality Drops.

Casey, A. (1994). *Kids Count Data Book*. Greenwich, Conn.: Annie C. Casey Foundation.

Governing. (1988). Infant Mortality: It's as American as Apple Pie. p. 50.

Healthy Companies. (1989). Babies and the Bottom Line.

Japan. (1951). *The Children's Charter*.

Raspberry, W. (10/16/89). Prenatal Care–For All Moms. *The Washington Post*.

Perinatal Loss:
Considerations in Social Work Practice

Carol K. Mahan, MSW
Judith Calica, AM, LCSW, BCD

SUMMARY. The death of a fetus or newborn infant prompts a grief response which has numerous unique aspects. Pregnancy losses are similar in many respects to other losses, but raise additional issues which require attention and consideration. This article addresses these issues, and offers guidance to social workers who are working with persons following this special type of loss. Parental communication, sibling needs and follow-up programs are also reviewed, along with caregiver issues. *[Article copies available for a fee from The Haworth Document Delivery Service: 1-800-342-9678. E-mail address: getinfo@haworth.com]*

For most parents, the birth of a newborn is an exciting, much anticipated event. The birth typically represents the fulfillment of a dream. Although not true in all cases (unwanted pregnancies in particular, and sometimes in unplanned pregnancies as well), for most parents the birth is considered a blessed or at least special event. Yet for a certain portion of pregnancies, dreams turn to nightmares when the pregnancy does not result in the birth of a healthy baby. Approximately 11 of every 1,000 babies born in the U.S. die in the neonatal period (Unicef, 1985). Further,

Carol K. Mahan is affiliated with Spirit Mountain Hospice, West Park Hospital, 707 Sheridan Avenue, Cody, WY 82414. Judith Calica is a Clinical Social Worker in private practice, 55 East Washington, Suite 1521, Chicago, IL 60602.

[Haworth co-indexing entry note]: "Perinatal Loss: Considerations in Social Work Practice." Mahan, Carol K., and Judith Calica. Co-published simultaneously in *Social Work in Health Care* (The Haworth Press, Inc.) Vol. 24, No. 3/4, 1997, pp. 141-152; and: *Fundamentals of Perinatal Social Work: A Guide for Clinical Practice with Women, Infants, and Families* (ed: Regina Furlong Lind, and Debra Honig Bachman) The Haworth Press, Inc., 1997, pp. 141-152. Single or multiple copies of this article are available for a fee from The Haworth Document Delivery Service [1-800-342-9678, 9:00 a.m. - 5:00 p.m. (EST). E-mail address: getinfo@haworth.com].

it is estimated that 10-15% or more of all pregnancies end in miscarriage. As a result, would-be-parents are faced with the grief that accompanies this particularly difficult loss. This article will address grief following perinatal loss, and will suggest intervention strategies for the perinatal social worker.

Researchers have known for some time that there are distinct patterns to the grief associated with death and other types of loss. Beginning in the late 1950s, medical journals began addressing grief, as well as the needs of dying patients. The topic came to the forefront for the general public with the publication of Elisabeth Kubler-Ross' classic book, *On Death and Dying* (Kubler-Ross, 1969). Her book marked the beginning of discussions among the general public, and remains an important work today. She, as well as other authors, discussed the reactions and stages associated with grief not only for the dying patient, but for his or her loved ones. The shock and denial which is felt immediately gives way to anger, depression and, eventually, an acceptance of the loss. However, despite enhanced awareness of grief, many people are unprepared for the enormity of emotion associated with death.

The realization that the death of a baby or fetus prompted a similar response did not come quite as quickly. Eventually, however, this special type of loss became the focus of researchers and health care practitioners caring for patients and family members in perinatal settings (Benfield et al., 1978; Engle, 1964; Kennell et al., 1970). Emotional support for parents and others has advanced greatly over the past two decades, as awareness of the special issues and needs of this population have become more widely recognized (Peppers & Knapp, 1980; Rowe et al., 1978; Kellner & Kirkley-Best, 1981; Lewis, 1979).

TYPES OF PERINATAL LOSSES

It is essential to consider the range of perinatal losses when developing support services for families. Types of losses include miscarriages, neonatal deaths, intrauterine fetal deaths (IUFD) and stillbirths. In addition, there are missed, elective and therapeutic abortions. Although not deaths, the failure to conceive and the birth of a child with medical problems or special needs are nonetheless losses associated with perinatal health care. These last two are outside the scope of this article, but are important to consider in the development of comprehensive programs addressing perinatal loss.

The others involve the death of an embryo, fetus or newborn infant. Each loss may result in a parental or family grief reaction. There are some aspects of each type of loss that make them unique; therefore, each will be briefly discussed.

Miscarriage: Despite the relatively common occurrence of miscarriages, the emotional pain which follows is quite difficult, and like most perinatal grief, often underestimated. Causality is often unknown. The ambivalence felt by many women in early pregnancy may contribute to feelings of guilt if the pregnancy ends in miscarriage.

The "missed abortion," in which the embryo has died, but a miscarriage has not begun when the problem is discovered, is frequently discovered on routine ultrasound. This adds the element of shock, as all was thought to be going well. The patient in this situation must decide how to proceed–to wait for bleeding to begin on its own, or to end the pregnancy with a D&C.

Miscarriages are difficult for all, but may be particularly so for couples who had difficulty conceiving, and had finally surpassed that hurdle. The same is true for couples who have experienced multiple miscarriages.

Therapeutic abortion: Some women learn of significant birth defects while still pregnant, and are offered the opportunity to terminate the pregnancy rather than carry the fetus to term. In some cases the child would live, but with handicaps, while in other situations the infant would not survive after birth. The process of decision making in such situations is difficult at best, and is often complicated by abortion politics and restrictions on second and third trimester abortions.

Elective abortion: Whether or not a perinatal social worker's place of employment actually performs elective abortions, the issues arise for social workers in perinatal settings. The politics of abortion, including availability, funding issues and pressure from involved and uninvolved persons are among the factors faced by women contemplating an elective abortion. Further, the lack of social acceptance of elective abortions prevents many women from seeking the support of others.

Intrauterine fetal death/stillbirth: These losses also involve unique issues. As the pregnancy has continued longer, there is typically greater attachment to the fetus, and comfort in having passed the "miscarriage stage." Preparations for the baby, such as readying the nursery, selecting names and arranging maternity leave are more likely to have begun, or even been completed.

Mothers experiencing these losses may question their attentiveness to their own body signals, such as decreased fetal movement, that might have warned them and possibly prevented such a tragedy.

The death of a baby immediately before or during the birth process is not only a shock, but truly a tragedy. There is usually little warning, and no reason to anticipate such a turn of events. Although less common now due to advances in fetal monitoring, for those parents affected by this loss the grief is enormous, and similar in many ways to the death of a neonate.

Neonatal death: The death of a newborn, whether premature or full term, incorporates additional issues which the family must face. One is consideration of pain the infant may have suffered during his or her short life. Parents in this situation are more likely to face treatment dilemmas, including discontinuation of treatment, which carry psychological burdens difficult for everyone. Lives may have been put on hold during the brief life of the newborn, which has implications for careers, relationships and finances.

Despite the varying circumstances, the commonalties in perinatal loss are striking. All relate to the failure to have the happy, healthy newborn that most parents anticipate. And in all of the above, there is a tendency on the part of the general public to underestimate the impact of the perinatal loss.

PRINCIPLES FOR SOCIAL WORK INTERVENTION

In any perinatal loss, the social worker is in a key and unique position to assist families with important tasks of grieving. Each member of the health care team plays an important role in assisting families at this critical time; however, the social worker, by virtue of training and responsibility within the perinatal setting, may be most able to assist the family with the difficult emotional issues they are facing. Services provided to the family may include crisis intervention, concrete services, information and referrals.

Chief among the perinatal social worker's responsibilities is facilitating the beginnings of a healthy, normal grief process. Some key principles which contribute to this are outlined below:

It is essential to provide families with the support and information to assist them in understanding what they are feeling, and what losing an infant or fetus will mean to them and their family.

It is inappropriate for the personal or religious beliefs or values of any member of the health care team to interfere with the family's right to grieve in their own way.

When presenting important information to parents, such as funeral options, it may be helpful if a support person is present. He or she can help the parents remember details otherwise easily forgotten or confused. However, one should always ask if it is acceptable to include another person, rather than assuming it is.

Emotional support of the family is essential. This does not mean, however, that the family should always have someone with them. It is important to offer time for parents, with or without extended family, to be alone with each other and with their baby.

As a result of the death, most families' abilities to process information and make decisions will be at least somewhat impaired. It will likely be helpful to limit information provided, to write down information that must be remembered and to not ask for decisions which can be postponed.

One of the most difficult tasks facing parents experiencing a perinatal loss is coping with the loss of someone they never really got to know. Some ways to help make the baby as real as possible include:

- Naming the baby: Although many parents do this anyway, some do not, especially in situations of therapeutic abortions, stillborn infants and miscarriages. A name helps add to the perception of the infant as an individual, and therefore an important part of the parents' lives.
- Seeing, touching and holding the baby: Most perinatal caregivers now recognize the importance of offering an opportunity to see, touch or hold a baby that has died (Mahan et al., 1981). There remains hesitancy among some caregivers in situations in which the baby or fetus is disfigured, especially when a pregnancy termination was involved. Families may take their cue from the social worker about what is appropriate. It is essential not to make assumptions about what is best for the family, but to explain all options. Seldom are the family's fantasies about the baby's appearance worse than the reality.
- Photographs: A photograph is appropriate to offer as a memento of the baby. Some parents only wish for pictures of living infants, while others are grateful for any visual remembrance of their baby. In situations of neonatal deaths, some parents may appreciate or even prefer additional pictures of the baby after death, as this may be the only time photographs could be taken without the invasive tubes and wires associated with neonatal intensive care.
- Tangible remembrances: Parents should be offered all tangible remembrances of the infant's brief life, including name tags,

armbands, hair which was shaved for IV's, blankets, certificates commemorating baptism or other rituals, etc.

In addition to the features present in any grief process, there are some additional issues faced by families when a fetus or baby has died. It will likely be helpful for families to know about these in advance, to avoid shock or alarm. For example, it is not uncommon for grieving parents to awaken at night, believing that they hear the baby crying in another room. Women whose baby died during pregnancy may still "feel" pregnant. Some report a sensation that feels like the baby kicking. Many families are preoccupied with the real or imagined image of the infant, and it is not uncommon to be preoccupied with fantasies of what might have been.

Before the family leaves the hospital or clinic (or when talking to them by telephone if they are not present), be certain to remind them to call *when*, not if, they have questions. This helps reinforce that all parents have questions.

FUNERALS AND MEMORIAL SERVICES

Most families have no experience in planning a funeral or memorial service, particularly for an infant. They may be unsure what is appropriate or possible in their particular circumstances. Religious and cultural beliefs will have an impact, so it is imperative that perinatal social workers become familiar with the traditions of the religious, cultural and ethnic groups served by their hospital or clinic. In addition, for social workers who work in obstetrical settings, it is important to become familiar with the applicable laws regarding the gestational age or weight at which formal arrangements must be made for a fetus who has died. Similarly, social workers in neonatal intensive care units must become familiar with the regulations and practices of their institution regarding donating an infant's body to science. Regardless of setting, it is important to be aware of the range of options available to families.

Most researchers and practitioners agree that some type of service commemorating the fetus or infant is an important part of the grief process. The gestation of the infant, circumstances of the loss, and personal beliefs of those involved will help determine what type of service is appropriate. Generally, the later in pregnancy the loss, the more formal the service is likely to be. Some families, having faced an early pregnancy loss such as a miscarriage, might choose an informal service in a place which is special to them, such as a park. They might read poems or speak informally about the miscarried fetus. Families who had a stillborn infant or neonate who died may choose a funeral in the more traditional sense. Infant funerals, although they incorporate many of the same aspects as funerals for older persons, are often simpler. There may be a shorter viewing/calling time, or only a graveside service. Some families may choose to hold their infant during a church or funeral home service.

Families, particularly those of limited means, will benefit from knowing that in most cases funerals for infants are far less expensive than funerals for older persons. It will be helpful for the social worker to direct families with limited means to sources of public assistance.

Because of their lack of experience with funerals and services, the family will likely rely heavily on information provided by the social worker. Although there is no clearly right or wrong way to proceed, it is an opportunity to encourage families to consider commemorating their child's existence in a way which will help, rather than hinder, the grief process.

CAUSALITY AND GUILT

Another issue which must be addressed with families facing perinatal loss is that of causality. Most parents are desperate for as much information as possible as to "what went wrong." Although information regarding causality is best shared by the physician members of the team, it is important for the social worker to be aware of the medical circumstances and of concerns the parents might have about the cause of their baby's death. Some parents worry endlessly–and unnecessarily–about minor events that are clearly not related, but are afraid to ask their doctor if their worries are founded. Their reluctance to try to verify the cause may stem from intimidation or a fear of appearing ignorant. It may also be a fear of learning that they were responsible for their baby's death. Most often, parents can be reassured that there was nothing they could have done differently to avoid the loss. Even if that is not the case, it is important to sensitively explore what concerns the family has regarding cause. Sometimes, parents did contribute to the pregnancy loss or baby's death. In such situations, the social worker can assist the family in sorting out their feelings of responsibility, and in learning from it for future pregnancies.

REACTIONS OF OTHERS

Despite the progress that has been made in understanding grief, many people still underestimate the impact of the loss of a baby. As a result, the reactions that parents receive from others may be insensitive. As with other aspects of the grief process, it may be helpful to prepare families in advance for reactions they may encounter. Some friends, relatives or co-workers may say nothing at all in response to the loss. Others may minimize the loss by telling parents "you can always have another baby," "at least you didn't get to know him" or "she probably wouldn't have been normal anyway." While these comments may be technically correct, they are unlikely to be of comfort to a grieving family.

PARENTAL COMMUNICATION

The death of a baby or fetus is an extremely painful experience for both parents. The grief process may be complicated by the differing needs and coping mechanisms of each partner. For example, one parent might wish to talk often and at length about the baby and his/her resulting grief, while the other does not want to discuss it at all. One parent might cry often, while the other shows no outward emotion. It is easy to understand how different styles of coping with grief can complicate a relationship. For mothers without a significant other involved, there may be even less support. Regardless of the nature of the relationship between parents, it is helpful to discuss the various ways each may cope with the loss. This knowledge may help prevent some problems, or encourage couples to talk together or to a professional about their different needs and ways of coping with the loss.

SIBLINGS

Other children of the family whose baby has died will be greatly affected by the death (Rosen & Cohen, 1981; Furlong & Black, 1984; Cain et al., 1964). For these families, there are additional issues which require consideration. What, when and how to tell the children? Most parents will appreciate guidance from the social worker.

In general, parents should be encouraged to be honest, but simple in discussions with their children. It is unnecessary to go into great detail with children, although parents will want to answer any questions they may have. Obviously, the amount and specificity of information shared with children must be appropriate to the developmental stage of the child. Many parents will want to incorporate their personal religious beliefs into the explanations that are offered children (e.g., the baby has gone to heaven, etc.).

There are a few classic mistakes that parents sometimes make in talking with their surviving children. It may be helpful to discuss these with parents. For example, parents are well advised never to use the expression "the baby went to sleep" when discussing death. Nor should they refer to the baby who died as having been "bad." It is also extremely important to explain that the baby's illness was not like the sicknesses that the other children get, lest the children develop fears that they, too, might die.

Some parents underestimate their child's awareness of this family crisis. While a toddler, for example, will not understand much about what is happening, he or she will likely be aware that something is amiss. It may be helpful to encourage parents not to hide the events which are occurring, as this may only heighten a child's fears.

FOLLOW-UP PROGRAMS

Whether highly structured or loosely organized, follow-up programs can provide an important link during the first few weeks or months following the death of an infant (Schreiner et al., 1979). Programs vary in timing and structure, but most have similar goals: assuring adequate information has been given to the family, assessing response to the loss and offering support during an emotionally difficult time. Hopefully, as a result, healthy adjustment to the loss will be more likely. Follow-up programs assist in the identification of grief which appears pathological, so that appropriate interventions and/or referrals can be made.

Follow-up programs are probably best organized in an interdisciplinary manner. Physicians and social workers can invite parents to return to the hospital or clinic a few weeks after the death to review the circumstances of the death, answer questions that parents may have about this and future pregnancies, review information about grieving and assess the parents' response to the loss of the baby. This is a good time to suggest that families wait several months before undertaking another pregnancy, to allow sufficient time for grief resolution (Pozanski, 1972).

It may also be helpful to provide or suggest reading materials. Although reading materials about fetal or infant loss will not be of interest to everyone, some parents find them helpful (Mahan et al., 1983). Bereavement support groups may also be a source of support for some families. This is a good time to share such resource information with parents, if it was not done earlier.

DISCONTINUING TREATMENT/PREGNANCY TERMINATION

There are circumstances associated with some pregnancies or births that add to the complexity of already difficult perinatal losses. These include, but are not limited to, decisions to seek elective or therapeutic abortions and decisions to discontinue treatment of critically ill newborns. Additional social work attention is appropriate, given to the added stressors families face in such situations. Religious, cultural and familial pressures may be present and may therefore complicate the decision-making process. Guilt and ambivalence may be greater factors than with other losses. The number of weeks gestation and other circumstances associated with the termination (distance the patient needs to travel to secure a second or third trimester therapeutic abortion, presence of anti-choice protesters, etc.) add both practical and emotional complications not only for the parents, but for everyone who is involved in these decisions.

When families are facing these difficult decisions, the social worker can help assure that pertinent issues are addressed, and that the family is able to consider all aspects of the decisions at hand. In some cases, an ethics committee may be involved, which may seem overwhelming to the family. The social worker can be instrumental in working with parents to enhance their understanding of, and participation in, whatever process a particular institution's bio-ethics committee utilizes.

CAREGIVER CONSIDERATIONS

Social workers hold it as a value to be available, compassionate and caring towards the families with whom they work. The opportunity to work with families facing a perinatal crisis is rewarding, and particularly in situations of perinatal loss, can contribute significantly to feelings of professional satisfaction when the social worker's therapeutic interventions contribute to a healthy grief process. However, the work is by nature also emotionally draining (Weinberg, 1990). Social workers with significant exposure to grief and loss would be wise to carefully consider their own issues related to grief and loss, and the meaning that working with grief holds for them.

Whether acknowledged or not, professionals working with grieving parents have unique, personal responses to each loss. Identifying the thoughts and feelings which exist, their meaning in the present and the memories they evoke, allows professionals to make conscious decisions about how to use these thoughts and feelings in a manner which is helpful for both the clients and the social worker. Too often, the personal responses of the worker are ignored, avoided, denied or the subject of disapproval. Acknowledging the feelings one has about grief work can help prevent "burnout" and enhance professional practice. However, to do so, one must openly reflect upon relevant personal experiences and values held about death and grief.

Repeated exposure to loss may not be emotionally healthy, particularly for persons whose personal losses were great, recent or remain unresolved. Repeated exposure can lead to professional "burnout," decreased sensitivity as a defense mechanism, or a skewed perspective about perinatal outcomes. One should be alert for signs that the stress of perinatal social work is interfering with professional or personal functioning. Preventatively, it may be helpful to participate in caregiver support groups; of mixed discipline perinatal health care staff, other hospital social workers or perinatal social workers from the surrounding community. If such formal mechanisms are not available, at a minimum the social worker might engage in discussions with a colleague or social work supervisor who faces similar issues or is understanding of them. Such opportunities allow the social worker to ventilate and process difficult cases, and to think through issues which may impact this important work. Other activities which might help include physical activity (to release tension), "mental health days" off from work and involvement in hobbies, volunteer work, etc., which are quite different from typical, high stress professional responsibilities.

Regardless of the specific techniques utilized to assure the emotional well-being of the caregiver, it is attention to this aspect of caregiving which is vital. An emotionally healthy social worker, who has worked through his/her own agenda and issues about death, will be much better able to assist grieving families.

Accepted for Publication: 05/14/96

REFERENCES

Benfield, D.G., Leib, S.A., Vollman, J.H. (1978) Grief response of parents to neonatal death and parent participation in deciding care. *Pediatrics*, 62, 171-177.

Cain, A.C., Fast, I., Erickson, M.E. (1964) Children's disturbed reaction to the death of a sibling. *American Journal of Orthopsychiatry*, 34, 741-752.

Engle, G.L. (1964) Grief and grieving. *American Journal of Nursing*, 64, 93-98.

Furlong, R.M., Black, R.B. (1984) Pregnancy termination for genetic indications: The impact on families. *Social Work in Health Care*, 10 (1), 17-34.

Kellner, K.R., Kirkley-Best, E. (1981) Perinatal mortality counseling programs for families who experience a stillbirth. *Death Education*, 5.

Kennell, J.H., Slyter, H., Klaus, M.H. (1970) The mourning response of parents to the death of a newborn infant. *New England Journal of Medicine*, 283, 344-349.

Kubler-Ross, E. (1969) *On death and dying*. New York: Macmillan.

Lewis, E. (1979) Mourning by the family after a stillbirth or neonatal death. *Archives of Diseases in Childhood*, 54, 303-306.

Mahan, C.K., Perez, R., Ratliff, M., Schreiner, R.L. (1981) Neonatal death: Parental evaluation of the NICU experience. *Issues in Comprehensive Pediatric Nursing*, 5.

Mahan, C.K., Schreiner, R.L., Green, M. (1983) Bibliotherapy: A tool to help parents mourn their infant's death. *Health and Social Work*, 8.

Peppers, L.G., Knapp, R.J. (1980) *Motherhood and mourning*. New York: Praeger.

Pozanski, E.D. (1972) The replacement child: Saga of unresolved parental grief. *Journal of Pediatrics*, 81, 1190-1193.

Rosen, H., Cohen, H.L. (1981) Children's reactions to sibling loss. *Clinical Social Work Journal*, 9 (3), 211-219.

Rowe, J., Clyman, R., Green, C. et al. (1978) Perinatal death. *Pediatrics*, 62 (2).

Schreiner, R.L., Gresham, E.L., Green, M. (1979) Physician's responsibility to parents after death of an infant. *American Journal of Diseases of Children*, 133, 723-725.

Unicef (1985) International infant mortality statistics.

Weinberg, I.J. (1990) Caring for the caregiver. *Bereavement*, 4 (4), 26-27.

SUGGESTED READINGS

Borg S, Lasker J: *When Pregnancy Fails*, Beacon Press, Boston, 1981.

Hales D, Johnson T: *Intensive Caring. New Hope for High-Risk Pregnancy*, Crown Publishers, Inc., New York, 1990.

Kushner HS: *When Bad Things Happen to Good People*, Schocken Books, New York, 1981.

Schiff H: *The Bereaved Parent*, Penguin Books, New York, 1977.

Stinson R, Stinson P: *The Long Dying of Baby Andrew*, Little, Brown and Co., Boston, 1983.

A Birth Father and Adoption
in the Perinatal Setting

Barbara J. Menard, MTS, MSW

SUMMARY. The role of the birth father in adoption is debated by lawyers, adoption professionals, and members of the adoption triad. At issue is how best to involve the birth father in the adoption plan while respecting the feelings of the birth mother, prospective adoptive couple, and rights of the child. This article examines emotional, legal and practice issues related to a birth father in adoption and implications for the perinatal social worker. *[Article copies available for a fee from The Haworth Document Delivery Service: 1-800-342-9678. E-mail address: getinfo@haworth.com]*

The rights of a birth father in the adoption process became the focus of media attention with the Illinois Supreme Court's decision in the Baby Richard case [*In re Adoption Petition of Doe*, 159 Ill. 2d 347, 202 Ill. Dec. 535, 638 N.E. 2d 181 (1994)]. Proponents of birth father rights hail the decision for expanding the role of the birth father in adoption (Ingrassia, 1993). Others express concern for the best interests of the child (Hollinger, 1993), and question the rights of the birth mother and adoptive parents.

The term birth father refers to the alleged natural father, biological, reputed or putative father of a child being placed for adoption. The husband of a woman who makes an adoption plan is considered by law to be

Barbara J. Menard is Birth Parent Counselor in Pregnancy, Parenting and Adoption Services at Catholic Charities in San Diego. She has served as Co-Chair of the Perinatal Social Worker Cluster in San Diego.

[Haworth co-indexing entry note]: "A Birth Father and Adoption in the Perinatal Setting." Menard, Barbara J. Co-published simultaneously in *Social Work in Health Care* (The Haworth Press, Inc.) Vol. 24, No. 3/4, 1997, pp. 153-163; and: *Fundamentals of Perinatal Social Work: A Guide for Clinical Practice with Women, Infants, and Families* (ed: Regina Furlong Lind, and Debra Honig Bachman) The Haworth Press, Inc., 1997, pp. 153-163. Single or multiple copies of this article are available for a fee from The Haworth Document Delivery Service [1-800-342-9678, 9:00 a.m. - 5:00 p.m. (EST). E-mail address: getinfo@haworth.com].

the presumed father, although he may not be the biological father. The impact of an adoption decision can be similar for both a presumed and an alleged father, and thus, the issues discussed can have application for both groups.

There are many concerns and varied feelings which may be experienced by a man named as an alleged or presumed father. There are issues regarding the relationship with the birth mother including the nature of the relationship, its current status, the way in which the birth father learned of the pregnancy, and his expectations for the relationship in the present and future. The birth father may have feelings about adoption in general, and about the placement of his child for adoption. He may be concerned about the selection of a prospective adoptive couple and his role in their selection. He may wish to meet or to establish a relationship with the adoptive couple.

This article will examine the issue of birth father involvement in the adoption process, specifically in a perinatal setting. A birth father is a significant part of the adoption triad with legal rights and responsibilities. He may offer support to the birth mother during labor and delivery, and possibly impact the life of the child. He may provide important medical and social history to the prospective adoptive couple. The birth father may have feelings of grief, loss, anger and depression, which require intervention. The increased practice of placing infants from the hospital directly with an adoptive couple gives perinatal social workers a unique opportunity to encourage the participation of the birth father in the adoption process and to offer appropriate interventions.

THE PROBLEM:
DEFINING THE BIRTH FATHER'S ROLE IN ADOPTION

There is a scarcity of literature addressing the role of the birth father in adoption, and the impact of an adoption decision on the birth father. Deykin et al. (1988) note that with the exception of teenage fathers, single fathers in general have not been included in research, and nothing is known about men whose newborn or infant children have been surrendered for adoption. They note that factors such as family pressures, a soured relationship with the birth mother, fiscal considerations and the negative attitude held by some adoption agencies all contribute to exclude the birth father from the adoption process and impact his feelings about the experience.

In examining the role of the birth father in adoption, one must begin by asking the question, who defines that role? Does the birth father himself take the lead in establishing his place in the adoption process? Is the role of the birth father dependent upon the relationship he has with the birth mother? Or does the birth mother decide how much involvement the birth father is to be allowed? Does the birth mother have the right to prohibit the birth father from seeing the infant? Do the wishes of the birth mother take precedence over the feelings of the birth father? Where does the adoptive couple enter into this process? Does a prospective adoptive couple have tme right to meet with the birth father against the wishes of the birth mother? Who helps the birth father process his feelings?

> Case: A single seventeen-year-old high school student is in labor supported by her mother and father. Her seventeen-year-old boyfriend, who is also present, has recently lost his job, and he and the mother realize their plan to parent the baby is not viable. The birth father/boyfriend reads profiles of prospective adoptive couples to the birth mother between her contractions. She moans, "Don't let this baby come yet, we haven't picked a couple."

The role of the birth father may be clearly defined in cases where the birth mother and birth father are in a positive relationship, and both believe that adoption is in the best interests of the child. They usually make decisions together and consult each other throughout the adoption process. They are both involved in the selection of the adoptive couple, in meeting and establishing a relationship with the couple and in signing papers relinquishing the infant. The Deykin study (1988) found that those fathers who were permitted to participate in the proceedings were more approving of adoption, while those who felt pressure for adoption from outside sources and felt excluded were opposed to adoption.

Schwartz (1986) writes that while birth fathers now have rights with respect to their children, their motives for parenting or blocking an adoption can vary. Pride in paternity or procreation may lead a father to see the child as his personal property, or property that must remain in his family, and thus, seek to block the adoption. Some men may seek custody in response to the absence of their own father, and the promise they made to themselves that they would never abandon their child like their father abandoned them. There may be cultural issues related to the birth father's decision to seek custody rather than allow his child to be placed for adoption.

> Case: An eighteen-year-old single pregnant college student reported that the birth father would take the baby to Mexico and have his mother raise the child rather than have her place the baby for adop-

tion. He would do anything including abduct the child rather than permit adoption.

Anger at the birth mother may be another motive for a birth father attempting to block the adoption plan. This may be especially true if the father wants to punish her for placing *his* child for adoption, viewing the decision as a personal rejection of him. Some birth fathers see a custody battle as a way of exercising power over others, especially the adoptive couple. A custody battle may be a means of gaining money or notoriety. The role of the birth father in opposing the adoption plan is determined by his feelings about himself, the birth mother and the meaning the adoption has for him.

Sachdev studied the attitudes of the members of the adoption triad toward the birth father's right of access to identifying information on adoptees. The birth father is more likely to become involved if the birth mother agrees to his involvement. Sachdev believes the birth mother should be encouraged to permit the birth father to participate in the decision-making process and states the birth mother may not recognize the father's needs for support and therapeutic help in dealing with his anxiety, remorse and emotional trauma.

This study reveals that with time the feelings of each member of the adoption triad, particularly the adoptees, changed in relation to the birth father. Greater involvement of birth fathers from the beginning of the adoption decision may contribute to an increase in their own positive feelings concerning the adoption. This involvement is likely to positively influence the feelings of the other members of the adoption triad.

THE BIRTH FATHER DURING LABOR AND DELIVERY

Case: A nineteen-year-old pregnant woman who has made an adoption plan goes into labor at 9 p.m. and arrives at the hospital accompanied by her boyfriend. Labor progresses slowly and around 3 a.m. a young man who is high on crystal and alcohol barges into the labor room demanding to see his baby, stating he is the father. The laboring woman asks him to leave. There are angry exchanges, and hospital security is called.

One of the issues related to the involvement of a birth father in adoption is the question, Should the birth father be present during labor and delivery? Who acts as the advocate for the birth father to ask if he has been included in the hospital plan? In conflictual relationships, who mediates between the birth mother and birth father to assure his role? What happens in cases like the scenario above when the birth father is a drug abuser, and the birth mother fears for her safety and that of the child?

There are occasions where the presence of the birth father in the labor and delivery room is a source of conflict and tension for the birth mother. However, in many situations, the participation of the birth father in labor and delivery can positively impact the relationships between the birth father, birth mother and adoptive couple, and can assist him in processing the adoption decision. A review of the literature on the role of fathers in labor and delivery seems to indicate that labor and childbirth can be a stressful experience for any man; that there is a progression of paternal behaviors after the birth of a child; that men can assume a variety of roles during labor and delivery; and that the roles are related to the interdependence of mother and father.

Westreich et al. (1991) found that the birth setting influenced the behavior of the father. Fathers assigned to a traditional setting were more involved in coaching breathing and gave more verbal encouragement to their partners than those assigned to a birth room. The structure of a traditional birth room and the assumption of traditional roles can enhance the birth experience for an involved birth father. This can increase the satisfaction of the birth mother, and positively impact the baby.

The progression of paternal behaviors of first time fathers with their baby immediately after birth was studied by Tomlinson et al. (1991). Their research indicated that fathers spend the majority of time in fairly passive activities or in distant behavior. These authors note that like the previous study, father-infant interaction can be influenced by the setting, and birth fathers less frequently engage in touch or movement with their infant, waiting until they were offered a chance to hold the infant. This study supports the fact that birth fathers do not interfere in the birth of their child, and usually wait until they are invited before they hold the newborn.

In a study of the feelings experienced by first-time fathers during labor and delivery, Nichols (1993) found that the behaviors fathers believed assisted the woman most during labor and delivery were primarily focused on helpful behaviors. Over half of all fathers listed "just being there" as one of the most useful things he did. This supports the value of the birth father's presence during labor and delivery to assist the birth mother, to form a connection with the baby, and thus, to positively impact their feelings about adoption.

Chapman (1991) examined the roles of coach, teammate or witness that fathers assume during labor and birth. Her research does not support the common belief that the majority of fathers desire to be coaches. The majority of men viewed themselves as witnesses who are present to provide emotional support to their partners and to witness the birth of their child. A birth father could be present at the birth of his child as a witness without engaging in an active role.

In a later study, Chapman (1992) noted that the degrees of mutuality and understanding within the couple's relationship were conditions that related to the type of role adopted by expectant fathers during labor and birth, and contributed to men's ability to meet the expectations of their partners. She concludes that expectant fathers experience labor and birth in their own way. There are a variety of roles that men can adopt during labor and birth. These roles are based on the man's personality, the couple's expectations of the experience, and the couple's relationship. She notes that couples need the opportunity to select a labor role that meets their unique patterns of interaction. This is particularly true for birth parents who may or may not be in an ongoing relationship, and have different feelings about the adoption plan.

THE LEGAL RIGHTS OF THE BIRTH FATHER

One of the most significant issues in the role of a birth father and adoption involves the question of his legal rights. A series of Supreme Court rulings and state statutes have defined the constitutional rights and the legal responsibilities and limits of the birth father in an adoption. Who advocates for the legal rights of the father in the adoption? At times the birth father must be challenged to recognize his rights and assume his responsibilities in a timely manner. Who helps a birth father to deal with his feelings after signing papers to legally relinquish a child for adoption?

> Cases: An alleged birth father signs a Denial of Paternity form and states, "I don't know if I am this baby's father. There were rumors that the mother was sleeping around. But I never knew my father, and I promised myself that all of my children would know their father. I can sign this paper, but I will always wonder if he is my child."
>
> A presumed father signs forms relinquishing the child that is not his, and reports, "I promised myself that no child of mine would be adopted. My mother had a son she placed for adoption before she married. We have never met him, but when anyone asks how many siblings I have, I always say eight and include him."

A review of the literature reveals that prior to the Supreme Court decision *Stanley v. Illinois* (1972), unwed fathers had no legal standing in court, and therefore, no legal rights regarding their newborn child and the birth mother's adoption plan. In *Stanley v. Illinois*, the Court ruled that the unwed father was entitled to a hearing on his fitness as a parent before his children could be removed from his custody under the due process and equal protection clauses of the Constitution.

This was followed by the case *Quilloin v. Walcott* (1978), where the Court upheld a Georgia statute that allowed a biological mother alone to consent to the adoption of her child if the biological father had not legitimated the child. The Court ruled that an adoption could take place without the unwed biological father's consent where he had never sought custody and the adoption did no more than legally recognize the existing situation of the child.

While the first ruling recognized the constitutional rights of birth fathers in adoption, the second ruling placed requirements and limits on the role of the birth father if he does not legitimate a child. Following this pattern, in 1979 the Court ruled in *Caban v. Mohammed* that a New York statute that required the unwed biological mother but not the unwed biological father to consent to the adoption of their children was unconstitutional when an unwed biological father's relationship to his child was "fully comparable" to that of the mother.

The ruling in *Lehr v. Robertson* (1982) further defined the responsibilities of the birth father. The Court declared that an unwed biological father's constitutional rights are a function of the actual responsibilities he accepts, and the "custodial, personal, or financial relationship" he develops for his offspring. The birth father has legal rights but these do not absent him from acting as a father.

Shanley (1995) notes that these decisions do not clarify whether under the Constitution an unwed biological father has a right to veto the adoption of a newborn even if he has had no opportunity to establish the kind of relationship and provide the kind of care that the Court has declared protects parental rights. Since the Court refused to hear the case of Baby Richard (*Baby Boy Janikova*), the Court has foregone the opportunity to resolve this issue. The landmark cases cited above have all involved the adoption of older children, not of an infant placed for adoption at birth.

In discussing the unwed father's legal right to know of his child's existence, Hamilton (1987-88) argues that nowhere is the protection of this right to know more critical than in cases in which a newborn infant whose existence is unknown to his/her father is surrendered for adoption by the child's mother. He expresses concern that the unknowing father forever loses every opportunity to experience the joys and heartaches of accompanying the child through life, and feels that this action would not be accepted or tolerated in any other context. He questions why the legal status of an unmarried male alters people's perceptions of the right to know.

State laws governing paternal consent to adoption vary widely. Some states seem to regard the unwed biological father as a "parent," and require his consent unless his rights are terminated. However, the states vary considerably in the evidence they deem sufficient for termination. "Recent Developments" (*Harvard Law Review*, 1991) discusses the New York Court of Appeals ruling *In re Raquel Marie X.* (1990) that an unwed father has a right to veto an adoption if he is willing to parent the child. The father must be willing to assume full custody, and not merely attempt to block the adoption. He must promptly manifest parental responsibility before and after the child's birth. This demonstration of responsibility should include: public acknowledgment of paternity; payment of pregnancy and birth expenses; steps taken to establish legal responsibility for the child; and other factors showing a commitment to the child.

Shoop (1994) discusses the California Supreme Court ruling *Adoption of Kelsey S.*, 823 P.2d 1216 (Cal.1992). The decision allows an unwed father to stop an adoption agreed to by the child's mother; "If an unwed father promptly comes forward and demonstrates a full commitment to his parental responsibilities, emotional, financial, and otherwise, his federal constitutional right to due process prohibits the termination of his parental relationship absent a showing of his unfitness as a parent." A father who has come forward can lose his rights only if a court finds him to be an unfit parent. Similar to the New York ruling, an unwed birth father can block an adoption plan if he has promptly acknowledged a child as his own, and demonstrates a full commitment to his parental responsibilities.

In a July 31, 1995 ruling [*Adoption of Michael H.*, 43 Cal.Rptr. 2d (Cal. 1995)], the California Supreme Court denied a birth father the right to block the adoption of his son because he did not demonstrate sufficient commitment to the child after learning of the birth mother's pregnancy. The Court extended the 1992 ruling by stating that "a father who wants to gain custody must demonstrate 'as full a commitment to his parental responsibilities as the biological mother allowed and the circumstances permitted within a short time after he learned or reasonably should have learned that the biological mother was pregnant with his child'" (Wilkins, 1995). In this ruling, the California Court seeks to clarify that the role of the birth father, like that of the birth mother, begins with pregnancy. It is not enough for the father to come forward after birth and block an adoption plan.

Drafting and applying statutory provisions to govern unwed biological parents' relationships to their offspring is difficult as noted by Shanley (1995). In her evaluation, lawmakers and judges must recognize that parental rights stem not only from biological and genetic ties, but also from lived relationships of care, nurture and responsibility.

> Legal and social discourse alike must put the lived relationship between parents and between parents and child, not the rights of individuals alone, at the center of the analysis of parental claims. In particular the language of a father's "right" to custody of his infant child based on his genetic tie obscures the complexity of the relationships involved in human reproductive activity.

Birth fathers do have legal rights in adoption. While states vary in the definition of these rights, current state court rulings have expanded paternity beyond biology to responsibilities that begin prior to birth.

IMPLICATIONS FOR PERINATAL SOCIAL WORKERS

This article has discussed issues related to a birth father and adoption including the emotional impact of the adoption decision on the life of a birth father, a birth father's involvement in labor and delivery, and the legal rights and responsibilities of a birth father.

The literature indicates that labor and birth can be a stressful experience for any man, and the adoption decision may heighten this stress for a birth father. Perinatal social workers offer support to all members of the adoption triad and need to encourage the birth father to assume the role that is most consistent with his personality, and that best reflects the level of mutuality and communication of the birth mother and birth father.

Social workers may need to act as an intermediary between the birth mother and birth father in relationships that are strained. It may be possible to engage the birth father as a witness to/presence with the baby, without his need to actively participate in labor and birth. The birth father can be encouraged to use gaze and proximity with the baby, which will enhance his sense of connection to the infant. This can help the father to own the baby as a reality, and to accept the adoption decision as a choice, and not something imposed on him by external forces.

Perinatal social workers need to be aware of the state laws regarding the legal rights of a birth father. They may need to counsel the birth mother against a hasty decision regarding placement of the child for adoption in order to circumvent the birth father's involvement. Perinatal social workers may need to challenge a birth mother to reveal all known information regarding a birth father in order to legally terminate his rights before the adoption can become final. Social workers may need to explain that the birth father has been accorded equal protection under the Constitution. However, the birth father needs to be challenged to demonstrate a commitment to a relationship with the child from the beginning of the pregnancy, and not seek to block an adoption after birth if he has not established a prior relationship.

Perhaps most difficult for the perinatal social worker is dealing with the emotional dimensions of the adoption decision for both the birth mother and birth father. These emotions may come spilling out in grief and sadness, in anger and hostility or in depression and denial. With every case the social worker will need sensitivity to the impact of the adoption decision on the birth father. A birth father may be fully involved in the adoption decision, birth and placement process, or may arrive to block the adoption decision, or may learn of the adoption decision only after he arrives at the hospital.

Whatever the circumstances of the case, the perinatal social worker must balance the varied needs and expectations of the client, usually the birth mother and child, with the needs of the birth father and the adoptive couple. As Sables (1994) discusses, adoption agencies need to implement programs that help the birth father, especially a teenage father, to become involved in the adoption process.

The decision to place a child for adoption is a major life event. The perinatal social worker is often present at a crucial moment for all the members of the adoption triad, the infant, the birth parents and the prospective adoptive couple. The perinatal social worker can be a significant figure in helping all members to be attentive to the birth event, to be aware of the legal and ethical dimensions of the adoption decision especially as related to the birth father and to be accepting of the wide range of feelings connected to the adoption decision. The impact of the adoptive placement for a birth father, and all members of the adoption triad, will be positively or negatively influenced by the knowledge, sensitivity, and quality of presence of the perinatal social worker.

Accepted for Publication: 05/15/96

REFERENCES

California Reporter 2nd Series, 43 Cal. Rptr 2d No.3, Sept. 1, 1995, 445-677.

Chapman, L.L. (1992). Expectant fathers' roles during labor and birth. *Journal of Obstetric, Gynecologic and Neonatal Nursing, 21* (2), 114-20.

Chapman, L.L. (1991). Searching: Expectant fathers' experiences during labor and birth. *Journal of Perinatal & Neonatal Nursing, 4* (4), 21-29.

Deykin, E.Y.; Patti, P.H.; & Ryan, J. (1988). Fathers of adopted children: A study of the impact of child surrender on birthfathers. *American Journal of Orthopsychiatry, 58* (2), 240-48.

Gitlin, H.J. (1995). "Baby richard" law poses many questions for adoption attorneys. *Chicago Daily Law Bulletin, June 19, 1995, 141* (119), 6 col.1.

Hamilton, J.R. (1987-88). The unwed father and the right to know of his child's existence. *Kentucky Law Journal, 76* (4), 949-1009.

Hollinger, J.H. (1993). A failed system is tearing kids apart. *National Law Journal, 15* (49), Mon., Aug. 9, 1993, 17-18.

Ingrassia, M. (1993). Standing up for fathers: The troubling case of baby jessica focuses attention on paternal rights in adoption. *Newsweek, 121* (18), May 3, 1993, 52-54.

Nichols, M.R. (1993). Paternal perspectives of the childbirth experience. *Maternal-Child Nursing Journal, 21* (3), 99-108.

Recent Developments: Family law–unwed fathers' rights–new york court of appeals mandates veto power over newborn's adoption for unwed father who demonstrates parental responsibility. (1991). *Harvard Law Review, 104* (3), 800-07.

Sables, D.K. (1994). Balancing fathers' and children's rights in adoption. Speech given at Catholic Charities National Pregnancy, Parenting, and Adoption Conference, Spokane, WA.

Sachdev, P. (1991). The birth father: A neglected element in the adoption equation. *Families in Society, 72* (3), 131-39.

Schwartz, L.L. (1986). Unwed fathers and adoption custody disputes. *American Journal of Family Therapy, 14* (4), 347-55.

Shanley, M.L. (1995). Unwed fathers' rights, adoption, and sex equality: Gender-neutrality and the perpetuation of patriarchy. *Columbia Law Review, 95* (1), 60-103.

Shoop, J.G. (1994). Some unwed fathers can block adoptions. *Trial, 28* (5), 14-16.

Tomlinson. P.S.; Rothenberg, M.A.; & Carver, L.D. (1991). Behavior interaction of fathers with infants and mothers in the immediate postpartum period. *Journal of Nurse-Midwifery, Midwifery, 36* (4), 232-9.

Westreich, R.; Spector-Dunsky, L.; Klein, M.; Papageorgiou, A.; Kramer, M.; & Gelfand, M. (1991). The influence of birth setting on the father's behavior toward his partner and infant. *Birth, 18* (4), 198-202.

Wilkens, J. (1995). Adoptive parents win in high court. *The San Diego Union-Tribune*, Tuesday, August 1, 1995, A-1, A-13.

Index

Note: Page numbers followed by t indicate tables.

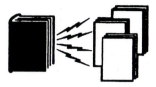

Haworth
DOCUMENT DELIVERY
SERVICE

This valuable service provides a single-article order form for any article from a Haworth journal.

- *Time Saving:* No running around from library to library to find a specific article.
- *Cost Effective:* All costs are kept down to a minimum.
- *Fast Delivery:* Choose from several options, including same-day FAX.
- *No Copyright Hassles:* You will be supplied by the original publisher.
- *Easy Payment:* Choose from several easy payment methods.

Open Accounts Welcome for ...
- Library Interlibrary Loan Departments
- Library Network/Consortia Wishing to Provide Single-Article Services
- Indexing/Abstracting Services with Single Article Provision Services
- Document Provision Brokers and Freelance Information Service Providers

---

MAIL or FAX THIS ENTIRE ORDER FORM TO:

Haworth Document Delivery Service
The Haworth Press, Inc.
10 Alice Street
Binghamton, NY 13904-1580

or FAX: 1-800-895-0582
or CALL: 1-800-342-9678
9am-5pm EST

PLEASE SEND ME PHOTOCOPIES OF THE FOLLOWING SINGLE ARTICLES:

1) Journal Title: _____
   Vol/Issue/Year: _____ Starting & Ending Pages: _____
   Article Title: _____

2) Journal Title: _____
   Vol/Issue/Year: _____ Starting & Ending Pages: _____
   Article Title: _____

3) Journal Title: _____
   Vol/Issue/Year: _____ Starting & Ending Pages: _____
   Article Title: _____

4) Journal Title: _____
   Vol/Issue/Year: _____ Starting & Ending Pages: _____
   Article Title: _____

(See other side for Costs and Payment Information)

COSTS: Please figure your cost to order quality copies of an article.

1. Set-up charge per article: $8.00
   ($8.00 × number of separate articles) _____
2. Photocopying charge for each article:

   1-10 pages: $1.00 _____

   11-19 pages: $3.00 _____

   20-29 pages: $5.00 _____

   30+ pages: $2.00/10 pages _____

3. Flexicover (optional): $2.00/article _____
4. Postage & Handling: US: $1.00 for the first article/

   $.50 each additional article _____

   Federal Express: $25.00 _____

   Outside US: $2.00 for first article/

   $.50 each additional article _____

5. Same-day FAX service: $.35 per page _____

GRAND TOTAL: _____

METHOD OF PAYMENT: (please check one)

❏ Check enclosed ❏ Please ship and bill. PO # _____
(sorry we can ship and bill to bookstores only! All others must pre-pay)

❏ Charge to my credit card: ❏ Visa; ❏ MasterCard; ❏ Discover;
❏ American Express;

Account Number:_____ Expiration date:_____

Signature: ✗_____

Name: _____ Institution: _____

Address: _____

_____

City: _____ State:_____ Zip:_____

Phone Number: _____ FAX Number: _____

MAIL or *FAX* THIS ENTIRE ORDER FORM TO:

Haworth Document Delivery Service   **or FAX:** 1-800-895-0582
The Haworth Press, Inc.   **or CALL:** 1-800-342-9678
10 Alice Street   9am-5pm EST)
Binghamton, NY 13904-1580